T0227248

Childhood Hearing Loss

Editors

NANCY M. YOUNG
ANNE MARIE THARPE

OTOLARYNGOLOGIC CLINICS OF NORTH AMERICA

www.oto.theclinics.com

Consulting Editor
SUJANA S. CHANDRASEKHAR

December 2021 • Volume 54 • Number 6

ELSEVIER

1600 John F. Kennedy Boulevard • Suite 1800 • Philadelphia, Pennsylvania, 19103-2899

http://www.oto.theclinics.com

OTOLARYNGOLOGIC CLINICS OF NORTH AMERICA Volume 54, Number 6
December 2021 ISSN 0030-6665, ISBN-13: 978-0-323-89744-0

Editor: Stacy Eastman
Developmental Editor: Diana Ang

Otolaryngologic Clinics of North America (ISSN 0030-6665) is published bimonthly by Elsevier, Inc., 360 Park Avenue South, New York, NY 10010-1710. Months of issue are February, April, June, August, October, and December. Business and Editorial Offices: 1600 John F. Kennedy Blvd., Suite 1800, Philadelphia, PA 19103-2899. Customer Service Office: 6277 Sea Harbor Drive, Orlando, FL 32887-4800. Periodicals postage paid at New York, NY and additional mailing offices. Subscription prices are $437.00 per year (US individuals), $1278.00 per year (US institutions), $100.00 per year (US & Canadian student/resident), $559.00 per year (Canadian individuals), $1348.00 per year (Canadian institutions), $610.00 per year (international individuals), $1348.00 per year (international institutions), $270.00 per year (international student/resident). Foreign air speed delivery is included in all *Clinics*' subscription prices. All prices are subject to change without notice. **POSTMASTER:** Send address changes to *Otolaryngologic Clinics of North America*, Elsevier Health Sciences Division, Subscription Customer Service, 3251 Riverport Lane, Maryland Heights, MO 63043. **Telephone: 1-800-654-2452 (U.S. and Canada); 314-447-8871 (outside U.S. and Canada). Fax: 314-447-8029. E-mail: journalscustomerservice-usa@elsevier.com (for print support); journalsonlinesupport-usa@elsevier.com (for online support).**

Reprints. For copies of 100 or more of articles in this publication, please contact the Commercial Reprints Department, Elsevier Inc., 360 Park Avenue South, New York, NY 10010-1710. Tel.: 212-633-3874; Fax: 212-633-3820; E-mail: reprints@elsevier.com.

Otolaryngologic Clinics of North America is also published in Spanish by McGraw-Hill Interamericana Editores S.A., P.O. Box 5-237, 06500 Mexico D.F., Mexico.

Otolaryngologic Clinics of North America is covered in *MEDLINE/PubMed (Index Medicus), Current Contents/Clinical Medicine, Excerpta Medica, BIOSIS, Science Citation Index,* and *ISI/BIOMED.*

Contributors

CONSULTING EDITOR

SUJANA S. CHANDRASEKHAR, MD, FACS, FAAOHNS
Past President, American Academy of Otolaryngology–Head and Neck Surgery,
Secretary-Treasurer, American Otological Society, Partner, ENT & Allergy Associates,
LLP, Clinical Professor, Department of Otolaryngology–Head and Neck Surgery, Zucker
School of Medicine at Hofstra-Northwell, Hempstead; Clinical Associate Professor,
Department of Otolaryngology–Head and Neck Surgery, Icahn School of Medicine at
Mount Sinai, New York, New York, USA

EDITORS

NANCY M. YOUNG, MD
Head, Section of Otology & Neurotology, Ann & Robert H. Children's Hospital of Chicago,
Lillian S. Wells Professor of Pediatric Otolaryngology, Northwestern University Feinberg
School of Medicine, Chicago, Illinois, USA

ANNE MARIE THARPE, PhD
Professor & Chair, Department of Hearing & Speech Sciences, Vanderbilt University
Medical Center, Nashville, Tennessee, USA

AUTHORS

FRED H. BESS, PhD
Department of Hearing & Speech Sciences, Vanderbilt University School of Medicine,
Vanderbilt Bill Wilkerson Center, Nashville, Tennessee, USA

CHRISTINE BROWN, AuD
Department of Hearing and Speech Sciences, Vanderbilt University Medical Center,
Nashville, Tennessee, USA

KEVIN D. BROWN, MD, PhD
Department of Otolaryngology Head and Neck Surgery, University of North Carolina at
Chapel Hill, North Carolina, USA

NICOLE E. CORBIN, AuD, PhD
University of Pittsburgh, Pittsburgh, Pennsylvania, USA

SHARON L. CUSHING, MD, MSc, FRCSC
Department of Otolaryngology, Head & Neck Surgery, Hospital for Sick Children; Archie's
Cochlear Implant Laboratory, Hospital for Sick Children; Department of Otolaryngology,
Head & Neck Surgery, University of Toronto; Institute of Medical Sciences, University of
Toronto, Toronto, Ontario, Canada

HILARY DAVIS, AuD
Department of Hearing & Speech Sciences, Vanderbilt University School of Medicine,
Vanderbilt Bill Wilkerson Center, Nashville, Tennessee, USA

RENÉ H. GIFFORD, PhD
Department of Hearing and Speech Sciences, Vanderbilt University Medical Center, Nashville, Tennessee, USA

SAMANTHA J. GUSTAFSON, AuD, PhD
University of Utah, Salt Lake City, Utah, USA

MELISSA HAZEN, Aud(C), MSc, HBSc
Department of Communication Disorders, Hospital for Sick Children; Archie's Cochlear Implant Laboratory, Hospital for Sick Children; Department of Otolaryngology, Head & Neck Surgery, University of Toronto, Toronto, Ontario, Canada

STEPHEN R. HOFF, MD
Assistant Professor, Department Otolaryngology–Head & Neck Surgery, Northwestern University Feinberg School of Medicine, Division of Otolaryngology–Head & Neck Surgery, Ann & Robert H. Lurie Children's Hospital of Chicago, Chicago, Illinois, USA

KIMBERLY HOLDEN, AuD
Ann and Robert H. Lurie Children's Hospital of Chicago, Chicago, Illinois, USA

LINDA J. HOOD, PhD
Professor, Department of Hearing and Speech Sciences, Vanderbilt University Medical Center, Nashville, Tennessee, USA

BENJAMIN W.Y. HORNSBY, PhD
Department of Hearing & Speech Sciences, Vanderbilt University School of Medicine, Vanderbilt Bill Wilkerson Center, Nashville, Tennessee, USA

CAROLYN M. JENKS, MD
Assistant Professor, Department Otolaryngology–Head & Neck Surgery, Johns Hopkins University School of Medicine, Baltimore, Maryland, USA

JUDITH E.C. LIEU, MD, MSPH
Professor, Department of Otolaryngology–Head and Neck Surgery Washington University School of Medicine in St. Louis, St. Louis, Missouri, USA

RYAN MCCREERY, PhD
Boys Town National Research Hospital

MARGARET McREDMOND, AuD
Vanderbilt University Medical Center, Nashville, Tennessee, USA

CALLI OBER MITCHELL, BS
Research Project Manager, Department of Obstetrics and Gynecology, Brigham and Women's Hospital, Boston, Massachusetts, USA

LEENA B. MITHAL, MD, MSCI
Assistant Professor, Department of Pediatrics, Division of Infectious Diseases, Northwestern University Feinberg School of Medicine, Ann & Robert H. Lurie Children's Hospital of Chicago, Chicago, Illinois, USA

CYNTHIA CASSON MORTON, PhD
Departments of Obstetrics and Gynecology and of Pathology, Kenneth J. Ryan, M.D. Distinguished Chair in Obstetrics and Gynecology and Director of Cytogenetics, Brigham and Women's Hospital, William Lambert Richardson Professor of Obstetrics, Gynecology and Reproductive Biology and Professor of Pathology, Harvard Medical School, Boston,

Massachusetts; Institute Member, Broad Institute of MIT and Harvard, Cambridge, Massachusetts, USA; Manchester Centre for Audiology and Deafness, School of Health Sciences, Chair in Auditory Genetics, University of Manchester, United Kingdom

LISA R. PARK, AuD
Department of Otolaryngology Head and Neck Surgery, University of North Carolina at Chapel Hill, North Carolina, USA

JOY RINGGER, AuD
Ann and Robert H. Lurie Children's Hospital of Chicago, Chicago, Illinois, USA

CAITLIN SAPP, PhD
University of Iowa, Iowa City, Iowa, USA

ANNE MORGAN SELLECK, MD
Department of Otolaryngology Head and Neck Surgery, University of North Carolina at Chapel Hill, North Carolina, USA

SAMPAT SINDHAR, MD, MSCI
Resident, Department of Otolaryngology–Head and Neck Surgery, Washington University School of Medicine in St. Louis, St. Louis, Missouri, USA

HILLARY SNAPP, AuD, PhD
Associate Professor, Department of Otolaryngology, University of Miami, Miami, Florida, USA

PETER S. STEYGER, PhD
Director, Translational Hearing Center, Biomedical Sciences, Creighton University, Omaha, Nebraska; Affiliate Investigator, National Center for Rehabilitative Auditory Research, VA Portland Health Care System, Oregon, USA

JENNA VOSS, PhD, CED, LSLS Cert AVEd
Associate Professor, Communication Disorders & Deaf Education, Fontbonne University, St. Louis, Missouri, USA

ELIZABETH WALKER, PhD
University of Iowa, Iowa City, Iowa, USA

KATHRYN WISEMAN, PhD
Boys Town National Research Hospital, Boys Town, Nebraska, USA

Contents

Compelling evidence indicates that some newborns harboring genetic variants associated with hearing loss will not be identified by current physiologic newborn hearing screening (NBHS) rendering current NBHS protocols suboptimal. Incorporating genomic sequencing into NBHS would improve clinical diagnosis and decrease time to early intervention efforts.

Patients with auditory neuropathy (AN)/auditory synaptopathy (AS) present unique evaluation and management challenges. Communication ability using auditory stimuli varies among patients, with particular difficulty understanding speech in noise. Auditory physiologic responses are key to accurate identification and monitoring of patients with AN/AS. Management approaches should consider individual variation and the possibility of change over time. Many patients with accurately characterized AN/AS demonstrate success with cochlear implants. Areas of discovery, including understanding of synaptic and neural mechanisms, genotype/phenotype relationships, and use of cochlear and cortical evoked potentials, will promote accurate clinical evaluation and management of infants, children, and adults with AN/AS.

Ototoxicity refers to damage to the inner ear that leads to functional hearing loss or vestibular disorders by selected pharmacotherapeutics as well as a variety of environmental exposures (eg, lead, cadmium, solvents). This article reviews the fundamental mechanisms underlying ototoxicity by clinically relevant, hospital-prescribed medications (ie, aminoglycoside antibiotics or cisplatin, as illustrative examples). Also reviewed are current strategies to prevent prescribed medication-induced ototoxicity, with several clinical or candidate interventional strategies being discussed.

> Children who are deaf/hard of hearing, including those from varied cultural and linguistic backgrounds, can use hearing technology to develop listening and spoken language successfully if given appropriate support. This is best accomplished by interprofessional teams providing caregivers with family-centered support from early intervention through the school-aged years. This approach is best practice because development of listening, spoken language, literacy, and social skills is most effective when caregivers are the primary communication partners and intervention agents, supported by qualified professionals. Special considerations are needed for families who have low access to services.

> There is mounting evidence to support the premise that children with hearing loss (CHL) are at increased risk for listening-related fatigue and its associated sequelae. This article provides an overview of the construct of listening-related fatigue in CHL, its importance, possible academic and psychosocial consequences, and recommendations for the identification and management of fatigue associated with pediatric hearing loss.

> Vestibular dysfunction is the most common comorbidity associated with childhood sensorineural hearing loss. Early identification of vestibular dysfunction enables early intervention to mitigate its impact of motor, behavioral, and neurocognitive deficits of developing children. Screening for vestibular impairment can be achieved in the busy clinical setting.

OTOLARYNGOLOGIC CLINICS
OF NORTH AMERICA

SERIES OF RELATED INTEREST

Facial Plastic Surgery Clinics
Available at: https://www.facialplastic.theclinics.com/

THE CLINICS ARE AVAILABLE ONLINE!
Access your subscription at:
www.theclinics.com

Foreword

The Importance of the Hearing, Language, and Educational Team in Addressing Childhood Hearing Loss

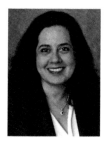

Sujana S. Chandrasekhar, MD, FACS, FAAOHNS
Consulting Editor

Childhood hearing loss includes that which is diagnosed shortly after birth using newborn hearing screening protocols, and that which is diagnosed later in childhood. The otolaryngologist who is alerted when hearing loss is identified in a child, no matter what age, must quickly assess the situation, determine what further testing is indicated and when, and counsel the parents using the latest information and resources. The hearing and language health team, including audiology, speech/language pathology, and otolaryngology, must work proactively with the parents/caregivers, the pediatrician, and the educators, to ensure the best speech, language, and learning outcomes for the child.

Drs Nancy Young and Anne Marie Tharpe have curated a thorough series of articles written by experienced, knowledgeable experts in this issue of *Otolaryngologic Clinics of North America* that the practicing Otolaryngologist can use as their handbook for understanding and managing childhood hearing loss. I congratulate Drs Young and Tharpe heartily on organizing the topics in a way that is logical and useful for otolaryngologists, audiologists, speech/language professionals, educators, pediatricians, and all others who interact with these children and families.

The reader is led through understanding of genetic issues relating to this condition, to mechanisms of identifying auditory neuropathy, to establishing hearing loss from ototoxicity and cytomegalovirus. We all need to understand guidelines and consensus statements to be able to implement evidence-based management. What are the right audiometric and medical tests to perform that yield the best assessments while minimizing discomfort to the child and their caregivers? When is vestibular evaluation

Otolaryngol Clin N Am 54 (2021) xiii–xiv
https://doi.org/10.1016/j.otc.2021.09.002
0030-6665/21/© 2021 Published by Elsevier Inc.

indicated, and what testing yields accurate information in children? These questions are answered by the article authors, enabling the treating team members to be logical and compassionate in their evaluation.

Once the evaluation is complete, when and how to intervene is the next hurdle to cross. The nuances of audiologic management for all degrees of hearing loss, and when to consider osseointegrated implants or cochlear implants are discussed in four comprehensive articles. And we do not assess or treat children in isolation. Paying attention to the family and school environment and knowing when to let up for a while are vital for the child's learning, emotional, and psychological well-being.

Congratulations again to Drs Young and Tharpe for their thoughtfulness in compiling the articles and choosing the authors for this issue of *Otolaryngologic Clinics of North America*. I encourage you, the reader, to savor each of these articles and share them with the other members of your team. Your patients and their families and communities will be the better for it.

Sujana S. Chandrasekhar, MD, FACS, FAAOHNS
Consulting Editor
Otolaryngologic Clinics of North America
Past President
American Academy of Otolaryngology–
Head and Neck Surgery
Secretary-Treasurer
American Otological Society
Partner, ENT & Allergy Associates LLP
18 East 48th Street, 2nd Floor
New York, NY 10017, USA

Clinical Professor, Department of Otolaryngology–
Head and Neck Surgery
Zucker School of Medicine at Hofstra-Northwell
Hempstead, NY, USA

Clinical Associate Professor
Department of Otolaryngology–
Head and Neck Surgery
Icahn School of Medicine at Mount Sinai
New York, NY, USA

E-mail address:
ssc@nyotology.com
www.ears.nyc

Preface

Current Perspectives on Childhood Hearing Loss

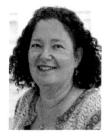 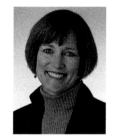

Nancy M. Young, MD   Anne Marie Tharpe, PhD
Editors

The demographics, diagnosis, and management of childhood hearing loss have significantly evolved since we, the editors, began our careers. Decades ago, we primarily served children with severe to profound hearing loss, typically the result of the rubella epidemic and genetic causes. Those children were usually identified at 2 to 2½ years of age and received limited benefit from hearing aids. Families' hopes for their children to develop spoken language were seldom realized, and many were educated in residential schools for the deaf. This issue of *Otolaryngologic Clinics of North America* provides an excellent review of the advances in care that have been achieved for children with hearing loss and their families today.

This issue begins with an article by Cynthia Morton and Callie Mitchell, summarizing remarkable advances in genetics of hearing loss. They make a compelling case for universal screening for genetic predisposition to hearing loss. Linda Hood clarifies current thinking about auditory neuropathy and its unique diagnostic and management challenges. Peter Steyger provides strategies to prevent medication-induced ototoxicity and presents a fascinating glimpse into future interventions for otoprotection. Congenital cytomegalovirus, the most common cause of nongenetic hearing loss and one associated with progressive loss, is summarized by Carolyn Jenks, Leena Mithal, and Stephen Hoff. They highlight the potential role of antiviral treatment when neonatal diagnosis is achieved.

Samantha Gustafson and Nicole Corbin provide a summary of a broad range of clinical practice guidelines to inform screening, diagnosis, and management of hearing loss in children. The authors point out the advantage of automated auditory brainstem response for newborn hearing screening, and the importance of timely management of otitis media and early cochlear implant referral. Joy Ringger, Kimberly Holden, and Margaret McRedmond emphasize the cross-check principle. This diagnostic approach combines the skills of behavioral testing with physiologic measures. The

Otolaryngol Clin N Am 54 (2021) xv–xvii
https://doi.org/10.1016/j.otc.2021.08.011
0030-6665/21/© 2021 Published by Elsevier Inc.

result is a powerful test battery more likely to yield an accurate diagnosis than any isolated test. Comprehensive management of children with hearing loss, including mild and unilateral loss, is eloquently covered by Kathryn Wiseman, Ryan McCreery, Elizabeth Walker, and Caitlin Sapp. The authors provide an evidence-based approach to comprehensive audiologic management to minimize the potential for developmental delays. Judith Lieu and Sampat Sindhar provide an excellent overview of medical evaluation of hearing loss that prioritizes reversible and treatable causes.

Rene Gifford and Christine Brown present a compelling case for expansion of cochlear implant candidacy so that children with bilateral hearing loss achieve better listening and language outcomes. Much clinical research, including results of their recent study, supports referral of children with unaided pure-tone average greater than 60 dB HL for implant evaluation. Lisa Park, Kevin Brown, and Anne Selleck summarize a new FDA-approved application of cochlear implants to unilateral and asymmetric hearing loss. The authors summarize studies demonstrating post-implantation improvements in speech perception, sound localization, and speech and language. The important topic of use of bone conduction devices, surgical and nonsurgical, in the pediatric population is illuminated by Hillary Snapp. Snapp provides a state-of-the-art review of the benefits, especially for children with aural atresia, as well as interventional challenges and limitations of this technology.

Jenna Voss elucidates the importance of a family-centered team approach by the multidisciplinary professionals supporting children using hearing technology. Voss highlights the benefit of involvement of a Certified Listening and Spoken Language Specialist on the team to promote auditory skills and spoken language development. The growing evidence that children with hearing loss are at risk for listening-related fatigue with negative academic and psychosocial consequences is provided by Benjamin Hornsby, Hilary Davis, and Fred Bess. The authors provide practical recommendations for identification and management of this important issue.

Vestibular dysfunction is the most common comorbidity associated with sensorineural hearing loss yet is rarely recognized or addressed. Sharon Cushing and co-author Melissa Hazen provide a practical and comprehensive approach to vestibular screening and an overview of the importance of its remediation.

The diagnosis and management of childhood hearing loss have improved considerably over the last several decades. The advances in hearing care, described in this issue, serve to remove many of the barriers to language development, educational outcomes, and quality of life once experienced by children with hearing loss and their families. Contemporary interdisciplinary support by otolaryngologists, audiologists, speech-language pathologists, and other professionals can ensure that children and their families achieve their desired and realistic goals.

Nancy M. Young, MD
Anne & Robert H. Lurie
Children's Hospital of Chicago
Division of Otolaryngology #25
225 East Chicago Avenue
Chicago, IL 60611, USA

Anne Marie Tharpe, PhD
Department of Hearing and Speech Sciences
Vanderbilt Bill Wilkerson Center
Vanderbilt University Medical Center
1215 21st Avenue South
Medical Center East
Nashville, TN 37232-8718, USA

E-mail addresses:
nyoung@luriechildrens.org (N.M. Young)
Anne.m.tharpe@vumc.org (A.M. Tharpe)

Genetics of Childhood Hearing Loss

Calli Ober Mitchell, BS[a], Cynthia Casson Morton, PhD[b,c,d,e],*

KEYWORDS

- Genomics • Genetics • Newborn hearing screening
- Single nucleotide variant interpretation • Copy number variant interpretation
- Precision medicine • Hereditary hearing loss • Early intervention

KEY POINTS

- Using genomic sequencing (GS), in addition to physiologic screening of audition, is a more effective approach to identify newborns having, and at risk to develop, hearing loss.
- The addition of GS to newborn hearing screening (NBHS) will optimize treatment and outcomes for infants and children with congenital hearing loss.
- GS provides beneficial etiologic information to families and clinicians.
- GS has the potential to decrease significantly the number of children lost to follow-up from NBHS and identify newborns with genetic hearing loss who pass NBHS due to nonpenetrance at birth.

INTRODUCTION

Hearing loss is recognized as the most common birth defect diagnosed in children in developed countries.[1] Permanent hearing loss creates challenges during development for individuals who are deaf and hard of hearing (DHH) and affects quality of life.[2] Early diagnosis and intervention have been shown to reduce developmental deficits among children who are DHH and financial burden on families, the education system, and health care systems.[3] For this reason, universal newborn hearing screening (NBHS) has been widely implemented in the United States for moderate-to-severe

[a] Department of Obstetrics and Gynecology, Brigham and Women's Hospital, NRB 160, 77 Avenue Louis Pasteur, Boston, MA 02115, USA; [b] Department of Obstetrics and Gynecology, Brigham and Women's Hospital, Harvard Medical School, NRB 160, 77 Avenue Louis Pasteur, Boston, MA 02115, USA; [c] Department of Pathology, Brigham and Women's Hospital, Harvard Medical School, Boston, MA, USA; [d] Broad Institute of MIT and Harvard, Cambridge, MA, USA; [e] Manchester Centre for Audiology and Deafness, School of Health Sciences, University of Manchester, UK
* Corresponding author. Department of Obstetrics and Gynecology, Brigham and Women's Hospital, Harvard Medical School, NRB 160, 77 Avenue Louis Pasteur, Boston, MA 02115.
E-mail address: cmorton@bwh.harvard.edu
Twitter: @CalliMitchell3 (C.O.M.); @CynthiaCMorton (C.C.M.)

Otolaryngol Clin N Am 54 (2021) 1081–1092
https://doi.org/10.1016/j.otc.2021.08.008
0030-6665/21/© 2021 Elsevier Inc. All rights reserved.

hearing loss since the Joint Committee of Infant Hearing endorsed NBHS in 1994.[4] According to the Centers for Disease Control and Prevention, greater than 98% of US newborns are screened for hearing loss and approximately 1.6 per 1000 screened newborns have some level of hearing loss.[5] By school age, this number increases to 3 to 4 children per 1000.[6] Childhood hearing loss is an etiologically heterogeneous trait with many recognized genetic and environmental causes.[6] **Fig. 1** shows the landscape of the causes contributing to childhood hearing loss diagnoses. Although injuries, infections, and exposure to excessive noise[7] can all contribute to development of hearing loss in children, between 50%[8] and 60%[6] of congenital and childhood hearing loss has a genetic origin,[9] and more than 1000 genes have been estimated to underlie hearing.[10]

GENETIC CAUSES OF CHILDHOOD HEARING LOSS

Genetic hearing loss can be categorized into 2 phenotypes: nonsyndromic and syndromic. Nonsyndromic sensorineural hearing loss is most commonly caused by autosomal recessive inheritance and accounts for at least 80% of congenital genetic hearing loss.[11] Syndromic hearing loss involves various other organ systems[12]—not uncommonly eye and kidney with varied modes of inheritance. Mitochondrial deafness is inherited through matrilineal relatives and is well

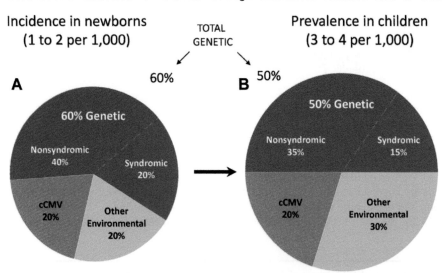

Fig. 1. Landscape of causes of DHH at birth and in childhood. (*A*) Incidence in newborns. Approximately 60% of congenital DHH is of genetic origin. Of genetic deafness, 30% is syndromic and 70% is nonsyndromic. Environmental factors contribute to 40% of congenital DHH diagnoses. As great as 20%[1,4] of environmental causes of deafness is attributed to congenital cytomegalovirus infections. Other environmental causes include prematurity, prenatal and postnatal infections, head trauma, subarachnoid hemorrhage, and pharmacologic ototoxicity.[6] (*B*) Prevalence in children. By childhood, the prevalance of DHH increases from 1 to 2 infants per 1000 to 3 to 4 children per 1000. Approximately 50% of DHH diagnosed in childhood is of genetic origin, and 20% is due to CMV infections. Other environmental factors including infections and structural anomalies contribute approximately 30%[8] of DHH. (*Adapted from* Morton CC, Nance WE. Newborn Hearing Screening — A Silent Revolution. *New England Journal of Medicine.* 2006;354(20):2151-2164. https://doi.org/10.1056/nejmra050700.)

recognized for genetic variants predisposing to ototoxicity from exposure to amino-glycosides.[13] Of note, some genes cause both syndromic and nonsyndromic deafness disorders and can display both autosomal dominant and autosomal recessive modes of inheritance.

SYNDROMIC HEARING LOSS

Hereditary forms of syndromic hearing loss are less prevalent than nonsyndromic forms.[9] Syndromic hearing loss has been associated with more than 400 syndromes, including Branchiootorenal syndrome, CHARGE syndrome, neurofibromatosis type 2, Stickler syndrome, Waardenburg syndrome, and Treacher Collins syndrome.[9,12] Pendred syndrome (PS), the most common autosomal recessive form of syndromic hearing loss, is caused by pathogenic variants in *SLC26A4* and affects between 7.5 and 10 individuals per 1000.[9] PS has been estimated to account for as much as 10% of hereditary deafness,[9] usually presenting as congenital severe-to-profound bilateral hearing loss. Pathogenic variants in *SLC26A4* are also the cause of a type of nonsyndromic autosomal recessive deafness (DFNB4).[9] Other common syndromes associated with autosomal recessive syndromic hearing loss are Jervell and Lange-Nielsen syndrome (prolonged QT syndrome), Usher syndrome, Perrault syndrome, biotinidase deficiency, and Refsum disease.[9,12]

NONSYNDROMIC HEARING LOSS

Nonsyndromic deafness is more prevalent than syndromic deafness, accounting for 70% of hereditary hearing loss.[9] Most of the genetic variants are missense and rare.[14] Consequently, 90% of DHH children are born into families without any history of hearing loss.[15] Approximately 15% to 20% of nonsyndromic hearing loss is inherited in an autosomal dominant pattern. X-linked and mitochondrial variations account for 1% to 1.5%, respectively.[11] To date, more than 50 autosomal dominant, more than 75 autosomal recessive, and 5 X-linked genes are known to cause nonsyndromic hearing loss[16] with more awaiting discovery. Current information and novel gene discoveries for hearing can be found on the Hereditary Hearing Loss homepage[16] (https://hereditaryhearingloss.org). Nomenclature for nonsyndromic genetic deafness is DFN (for deafness), followed by an A (dominant) or B (recessive), and a consecutive number based on order of discovery. X-linked deafness is designated as DFN followed by an X and an ascending number for its sequence in identification.

AUTOSOMAL RECESSIVE NONSYNDROMIC HEARING LOSS

Autosomal recessive nonsyndromic hearing loss usually presents prelingually and results in severe-to-profound hearing loss. Accounting for up to 50% of diagnoses,[17] the most prominent cause of severe-to-profound autosomal recessive hearing loss in most populations is caused by *GJB2* (DFNB1) variants.[18] Pathogenic variants in *SLC26A4* (DFNB4) are the second most common cause of autosomal recessive hearing loss and can also cause syndromic hearing loss in Pendred syndrome, manifesting with enlarged vestibular aqueducts.[9,12,17] Variants in *STRC* (DFNB16) are a major contributor of mild-to-moderate autosomal recessive nonsyndromic hearing loss.[18] Identification of hearing loss due to *STRC* variants is clinically relevant, as contiguous deletions can affect the *CATSPER2* gene nearby and cause Deafness Infertility syndrome in men. Because of repeated DNA segments at the locus, *STRC* is predisposed to copy number variants (CNVs),[9] which complicates variant interpretation.

AUTOSOMAL DOMINANT HEARING LOSS

Frequently, autosomal dominant hearing loss is postlingual, progressive, and milder than recessive forms.[9] Unlike autosomal recessive hearing loss where *GJB2 and SLC26A4* are the most prevalent causes, in autosomal dominant hearing loss there is no single gene that accounts for a significant proportion of etiologic diagnoses.[17] Pathogenic variants in *COCH* (DFNA9), *KCNQ4* (DFNA2), *DFNA5,* and *POU4F3* (DFNA16) are associated with high-frequency hearing loss.[9] Other autosomal dominant pathogenic variants cause mid-frequency deficits such as *TECTA* (DFNA8/12) and *COL11A2* (DFNA13) and low-frequency deficits with *WFS1* (DFNA6/14/38).[9,17]

SEX CHROMOSOME–LINKED HEARING LOSS

To date, 5 X-linked genes have been associated with hearing loss with the most common due to variants in *POU3F4* (DFNX2).[9,17] Pathogenic variants in *COL4A5* cause Alport syndrome, a syndromic form of X-linked hearing loss with kidney pathology that usually presents late in childhood.[9] Another X-linked syndromic form is Mohr-Tranebjærg syndrome caused by genetic variants in *TIMM8A*.[9] Only one locus to date has been assigned to the Y chromosome, DFNY1, discovered in 2004 in a large Chinese family and caused by an insertion of chromosome 1 DNA sequence into the Y chromosome.[19] DFNY1 has also been observed in one other Chinese family presenting with similar audiologic characteristics.[19]

MITOCHONDRIAL HEARING LOSS

Mitochondrial diseases most often involve multiple organ systems, and syndromic hearing loss is present in approximately 70% of affected individuals.[9] MELAS (mitochondrial encephalopathy, lactic acidosis, and strokelike episodes) syndrome, MERRF (myoclonic epilepsy with ragged-red fibers syndrome, Kearns-Sayre syndrome, and MIDD (maternally inherited diabetes and deafness) result in mitochondrial hearing loss.[9] One common nonsyndromic form of mitochondrial deafness is due to a variant in the mitochondrial 12S ribosomal ribonucleic acid gene. This variant, A1555G, has been estimated to be present in as many as 1 in 500 Caucasians.[17] Individuals with this variant are at risk to develop severe hearing loss from exposure to ototoxic aminoglycosides.[20] Maternal relatives harboring *MT-RNR1* variants are susceptible to ototoxicity given mitochondrial maternal inheritance and should avoid aminoglycoside antibiotics.[13] The PALOH (Pharmacogenetics to Avoid Loss of Hearing) study conducted recently in the United Kingdom implemented point-of-care genetic testing to intervene with potential ototoxicity in infants being treated in the neonatal intensive care unit. This study found that incorporating genetic testing in time sensitive, acute situations could avoid as many as 180 cases of aminoglycoside-induced ototoxicity in the United Kingdom each year.[21]

DISCUSSION

Precision medicine offers personalized treatments for individuals using their genetic information. With more than 15 countries currently providing novel genomic sequencing projects[22] since the completion of the Human Genome Project in 2003, an appreciation for the impact of molecular genomics on disease frequency has enabled implementation of genomics in diagnostic care. Personalized therapeutics and interventions can be developed using information from *genome sequencing* that encompasses assessing variants in all of an individual's 3×10^9 base pairs of DNA, *exome sequencing* that provides DNA sequence of 1% to 2% of the genome encoding proteins, or *gene panels* of selected genes of interest relevant to the condition under study. Advancements made in the past 2 decades have facilitated rapid and low-cost diagnostics for patients with hearing loss.[7] Today, various genetic panels are used in the diagnosis of congenital and childhood hearing loss. These panels, spanning from 23 to 252 genes,[1] provide assessment of genes associated with inheritance patterns of autosomal dominant, autosomal recessive, X-linked and mitochondrial deafness, and syndromic and nonsyndromic forms.

HEARING IN GENERATION GENOME: COMPREHENSIVE NEWBORN HEARING SCREENING

Before implementation of next-generation sequencing (NGS), most diagnostic laboratories analyzed a limited number of hearing loss genes, beginning with *GJB2* given its high prevalence among DHH individuals and yielding a diagnosis in about 10% to 20% of cases.[23] In recent years, advances in gene discovery and analysis increased the diagnostic yield range from 39%[18] to 50%.[24] A recent review reports that using congenital cytomegalovirus (cCMV) analysis and targeted NGS panels for hearing loss has increased the diagnostic yield for congenital bilateral loss to 77.9%,[25] depending on the DHH population being studied.

Determining the cause of a child's hearing loss can provide prognostic information as well as predict the chance of familial reoccurrence.[9] Studies have described the benefits of using genetic testing as a prognostic tool, such as the outcome performance shown by cochlear implant recipients with *GJB2* and *SLC26A4* related deafness.[26,27] In 2002, Green and colleagues[26] found that effective rehabilitation is possible for individuals with profound hearing loss due to *GJB2* deafness through cochlear implantation. More recent data provide further insight into benefits of cochlear implantation in a variety of deafness-causing genes including *GJB2*, *SLC26A4*, *OTOF*, *CACNA1D*, *CABP2*, *SLC17A8*, *DIAPH3*, *OPA1*, and *ROR1*.[28] Using genetic testing to predict cochlear implant outcomes will lead to better clinical management for individuals with genetic deafness.[29]

The prevalence of hearing loss continues to increase in childhood up to school age.[6] An explanation for this is, in part at least, because of limitations of current NBHS practices. Although NBHS is often successful in identifying infants with congenital hearing loss, it does not adequately detect mild or delayed onset loss or children with auditory neuropathy and has a high false-positive rate[4] and high loss-to-follow-up rate in the United States (~26% for recent data[5,30]). By implementing genomic sequencing (GS) into NBHS, Wang and colleagues found a decrease in the loss-to- follow-up rate among families with a genetic cause.[13] Shearer and colleagues proposed comprehensive NBHS with the addition of genetic testing and cCMV testing alongside standard physiologic NBHS. Including genomic sequencing in NBHS would identify newborns with genetic hearing loss missed on physiologic NBHS, allowing for a comprehensive analysis of causes including common genes known to cause hearing loss and viral infections such as cCMV.[4] Comprehensive NBHS would lead to improved diagnostic yields, earlier intervention, and thus, better outcomes for DHH babies and children.

SEQaBOO (SEQuencing A BABY FOR AN OPTIMAL OUTCOME): GENOME SEQUENCING FOR NEWBORN SCREEN

A study initiated in Boston, Massachusetts, SEQaBOO (SEQuencing a Baby for an Optimal Outcome), aims to identify genetic variants for deafness and be at the forefront of precision medicine treatments for newborns and children who are DHH.

Participants are recruited from 3 Harvard Medical School affiliated hospitals: Brigham and Women's Hospital (BWH), Boston Children's Hospital (BCH), and the Massachusetts Eye and Ear (MEE). Parents and newborns referred following a positive NBHS at BWH or at confirmatory diagnostic audiometry at BCH or MEE can elect to receive comprehensive genomic sequencing and interpretation of curated genes for hearing loss. Parents can additionally obtain ACMG v3.0 secondary findings for themselves. ACMG v3.0 secondary genes are a group of 73 genes proposed by the American College of Medical Genetics and Genomics[31] for which an individual might pursue some intervention, were it to be discovered that a pathogenic variant was present (eg, colonoscopy at an earlier age than otherwise recommended). Alternatively, parents can enroll only for annual surveys administered to all participating families to ascertain evolving attitudes on genomic testing in addition to family medical history and health information.

SEQaBOO MANCHESTER: PANEL TESTING AVAILABLE THROUGH THE NATIONAL HEALTH SERVICE

Running in parallel, SEQaBOO Manchester, England plans to use the National Health Service (NHS) hearing loss panel that reports on 115 genes associated with hearing loss. This panel was introduced in April 2021 to parents of newborns identified to have hearing loss by the national newborn hearing screening program. Approval to begin recruitment at 4 Manchester University NHS Trust hospitals has been granted. Parents who enroll in SEQaBOO Manchester will take part in annual surveys aimed at assessing evolving attitudes and opinions on genomic testing in addition to family medical history and health information.

IMPLICATIONS OF CURRENT PHYSIOLOGIC NEWBORN HEARING SCREENING

Since implementation of NBHS in the 1990s, many children who are DHH were discovered at a much earlier age than would have occurred without NBHS, allowing for timely interventions. However, NBHS is not designed to identify all infants who are at risk for hearing loss. For example, infants with normal or mild hearing loss at birth might develop delayed onset or progressive hearing loss not identified by current physiologic NBHS approaches.

Given the extreme heterogeneity of hearing loss, current NBHS is ineffective in as many as 25% to 50%[13,32–35] of positive genetic cases because they pass contemporary NBHS. Screening a limited number of the most common variants in *GJB2* and *SLC26A4* has shown to benefit detection of DHH individuals. Genetic screening would be a valuable adjunctive screen to current physiologic NBHS. In a study of 180,469 neonates in Beijing, China using concurrent hearing and genetic screening, Dai and colleagues[32] found 9 neonates with etiologic variants in *GJB2* and 1 with a homozygous pathogenic variant in *SLC26A4* who passed both initial and secondary hearing screens (**Table 1**). Further follow-up indicated 9 of the children suffered from varying degrees of hearing loss (mild to severe), suggesting that approximately 27% of infants with pathogenic combinations of *GJB2* variants and about 14% of infants with pathogenic combinations of *SLC26A4* variants will pass NBHS and most of them will develop hearing loss by age 5 years.[32] **Fig. 2** shows the approximate 27% of DHH individuals harboring biallelic variants in *GJB2* who are not likely to be identified using current physiologic NBHS.

Another study in China analyzed 1,172,504 newborns and found that incorporating genetic testing into NBHS leads to an increase in detection rate of 13%[13] by 3 months of age. Notably, of the positive genetic cases, 42% would not benefit from physiologic

Table 1
Pathogenic variants for DHH nonpenetrant on functional newborn hearing screening

Newborn	Gene	Variants	Phenotype of DHH
1.	GJB2	c.299delAT/c.299delAT	Mild/severe bilateral
2.	GJB2	c.235delC/c.235delC	Lost to follow-up
3.	GJB2	c.176del16/c.235delC	Moderate bilateral
4.	GJB2	c.235delC/c.299delAT	Severe bilateral
5.	GJB2	c.235delC/c.299delAT	Moderate bilateral
6.	GJB2	c.235delC/c.235delC	Moderate bilateral
7.	GJB2	c.235delC/c.299delAT	Mild bilateral
8.	GJB2	c.235delC/c.235delC	Moderate bilateral
9.	GJB2	c.235delC/c.235delC	Moderate bilateral
10.	SLC26A4	c.919A>G/c.919A>G	Mild unilateral

Data obtained from Dai and co-authors in concurrent hearing and genetic screening study[32]; 10 neonates with pathogenic variants in GJB2 and SLC26A4 passed newborn hearing screening and nine were confirmed to be DHH with one lost to follow up.

NBHS alone. Wang and colleagues highlight the improvement in diagnostic yield allowing for earlier interventions and better outcomes by using concurrent genetic testing along with physiologic NBHS.[13] These data are consistent with other studies; for example, Guo and colleagues[35] found that 31% of individuals with positive genetic results passed NBHS. An earlier study by Minami and colleagues[34] suggests that the number of individuals who are DHH and harbor biallelic GJB2 variants nonpenetrant on NBHS is much larger than that reported in previous studies; their study found 57% of patients with biallelic GJB2 variants passed NBHS to be diagnosed later as DHH. Wu and colleagues also noted a large percentage of newborns passing NBHS, with 56.1%[33] of newborns having conclusive genetic diagnoses for their

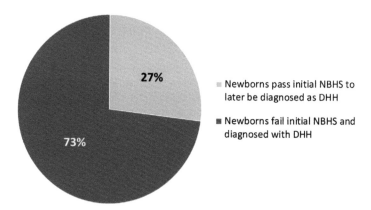

27%

73%

- Newborns pass initial NBHS to later be diagnosed as DHH
- Newborns fail initial NBHS and diagnosed with DHH

Fig. 2. Percentage of newborns harboring etiologic pathogenic GJB2 variants. This chart highlights the percentage of newborns harboring etiologic pathogenic GJB2 variants that will be missed by standard NBHS alone. These data obtained from Dai and colleagues[32] demonstrate the importance of concurrent hearing and genetic screening in newborns to yield the highest diagnostic rate for DHH individuals. Nine of thirty-three newborns harboring etiologic GJB2 variants passed the initial hearing screen and later were diagnosed as DHH.

hearing loss. These data indicate the need to implement universal genetic testing for such variants that are likely to be missed on standard NBHS.

A recent initiative in Victoria, Australia using the platform of the Victorian Childhood Hearing Impairment Longitudinal Databank, which provides natural history data on development and resource use for DHH, translation of genetic findings can be accomplished to improve care for DHH children. Through this platform, the Melbourne Genomics Health Alliance offered targeted exome sequencing.[36] A population cohort of bilateral moderate, severe, or profound hearing loss was recruited to join the Baby Beyond Hearing Project.[37] Of 106 infants who underwent genetic testing, 56% received a diagnosis, with 21% harboring pathogenic variants in GJB2 or GJB6.[37] The most common causative genes in addition to GJB2 were SLC26A4 (5%), MYO15A (5%), and STRC (4%).[38] Downie and colleagues found that 81% of diagnoses were inherited in an autosomal recessive pattern. As part of a larger aim of the study, analyzing parents' opinions and the psychosocial impact of offering additional findings for their newborns, the investigators noted that personal values and circumstances affected the level of information parents seek to obtain from genomic sequencing.[37,39] A cost-effectiveness analysis was completed on this cohort of DHH individuals that provides evidence that genetic testing is valuable at preventing further investigation and creating more efficient and timely clinical management.[40]

As part of Ontario's Infant Hearing Program, hearing loss risk factor screening was initiated into universal NBHS in July 2019. Dried blood spots are screened for cCMV and variants in GJB2, GJB6, and SLC26A4[41,42] to identify DHH individuals early to limit scenarios where DHH children go undetected by current physiologic NBHS methods. More children are identified and provided with services earlier due to recognition of genetic and environmental causes leading to improved understanding of cause and improved surveillance mechanisms. For example, using dried blood spots enabled risk factor screening to proceed during the COVID-19 pandemic when standard NBHS was suspended ensuring that fewer DHH newborns were missed. Knowing the genotype allows for surveillance for screen positives with genetic variants to be monitored for developing hearing loss later during childhood[43] (information obtained via personal communication with Marie Pigeon).

COPY NUMBER VARIANT ANALYSIS IS ESSENTIAL IN DETERMINING ETIOLOGIC DIAGNOSES FOR GENETIC HEARING LOSS

Copy number variation is a large source of variation in the human genome, resulting in a 1.2% difference in comparison to the reference genome.[44] Previous studies have reported the importance of incorporating CNV analysis into genomic interpretation for efficient diagnosis of cause of childhood and congenital hearing loss.[45] CNVs are causal or contributory for an etiologic diagnosis in greater than 15% of DHH individuals.[18,44,45] More than 20 genes for hearing have been identified to have copy number deletions or duplications,[45] indicating the powerful influence of CNV detection in genetic hearing loss diagnoses. **Table 2** highlights the most prevalent hearing loss–associated genes with known CNVs.

COMPREHENSIVE NEWBORN HEARING SCREENING INCLUDES CONGENITAL CYTOMEGALOVIRUS ANALYSIS

In developed countries, cytomegalovirus is the most common intrauterine virus[46] with a highly variable presentation, and many newborns are asymptomatic. cCMV is the most common nongenetic cause of hearing loss,[23] and approximately 10% of otherwise asymptomatic cCMV cases develop congenital hearing loss.[46] Estimates

Table 2	
Most prevalent DHH genes identified with copy number variants[45]	
Gene	**Phenotype**
STRC	ARNSHL, deafness infertility syndrome (DIS)
OTOA	ARNSHL
GJB2	ARNSHL, ADNSHL
GJB6	ARNSHL, ADNSHL
SLC26A4	ARNSHL, Pendred syndrome (PS)
PCDH15	ARNSHL, Usher syndrome type 1F (USH1F)
POU3F4	XLNSHL
TMC1	ARNSHL

Data from Shearer AE, Kolbe DL, Azaiez H, et al. Copy number variants are a common cause of non-syndromic hearing loss. Genome Medicine. 2014;6(5):0-9. doi:10.1186/gm554.

indicate that 15% to 20% of childhood hearing loss can be attributed to cCMV infections.[1,4] Testing for cCMV must be performed before 3 weeks of age due to the abundance of CMV the environment.

SUMMARY

Recent compelling data in support of genetic diagnoses in newborns with congenital hearing loss or in DHH babies nonpenetrant at birth are well recognized for timely optimal developmental outcomes.[25,32] A comprehensive NBHS program including testing for pathogenetic variants and cCMV infection in addition to physiologic screening is technically feasible to implement. Initiatives such as those implemented in Australia, China, Taiwan, England, and Canada have demonstrated comprehensive NBHS is achievable and leads to improved outcomes for DHH individuals and their families.

FUTURE DIRECTIONS

A study conducted by Raymond and colleagues at Egleston Children's Hospital of Children's Healthcare of Atlanta analyzing genetic testing for congenital SNHL found that although genetics is the main cause, genetic testing or consultation was not uniformly ordered in the cohort.[47] Through early detection and intervention, delayed speech and language development are improved[48] but comprehensive NBHS must be incorporated into routine medical care.

Increasing access and affordability to GS has led to identification of novel human variants and better clinical management of individuals with hearing loss. Further research is needed to improve the knowledge of underlying pathology of these genetic variants. Through utilization of animal models or patient-derived cells, appropriate therapeutic and restorative approaches[49] are on the horizon, making it increasingly important to understand and identify the genetic causes of hearing loss. Currently more than 43 companies are focused on developing novel therapeutics for inner ear and central hearing disorders.[50] Comprehensive NBHS including physiologic testing, genetic testing, and cCMV testing can prevent unnecessary treatments such as antiviral drugs for cCMV infections[46] or aminoglycosides for individuals with a genetic predisposition for ototoxicity.[20,21] Newborn screening has long been driven by technology and can now embrace integration of genetic testing to provide life-altering treatments and management for individuals who are DHH.

CLINICS CARE POINTS

- A signficant number of children who pass NBHS have progressive losses or develop delayed onset of sensorineural hearing loss. Newborn screening needs to include genetic testing to identify newborns with genetic variants with risk to develop nonpenetrant hearing loss at birth.
- Testing for a limited number of genetic variants as part of newborn screening for all children can identify 50% of children expected to have delayed onset of hearing loss.
- Knowledge of mitochondrial genetic variants such as m.A1555G can be used in preventing hearing loss.
- Identification of cCMV can lead to early treatment that, in some cases, halts progression of hearing loss.

ACKNOWLEDGMENTS

C.C. Morton acknowledges support by the National Institutes of Deafness and Other Communication Disorders, National Institutes of Health (DC015052) and also support by the NIHR Manchester Biomedical Research Centre.

DISCLOSURE

The authors have no disclosures to report.

REFERENCES

1. Thorpe RK, Smith RJH. Future directions for screening and treatment in congenital hearing loss. Precision Clin Med 2020;3(3):175–86.
2. Lindburg M, Ead B, Jeffe DB, et al. Hearing loss–related issues affecting quality of life in preschool children. Otolaryngol Head Neck Surg 2021;164(6):1322–9.
3. Krug E, Cieza A, Chadha S, et al. Childhood hearing loss strategies for prevention and care 2016. Available at: http://www.who.int/about/licensing/copyright_form/index.html. Accessed June 29, 2021.
4. Shearer AE, Shen J, Amr S, et al. A proposal for comprehensive newborn hearing screening to improve identification of deaf and hard-of-hearing children. Genet Med 2019;21(11):2614–30.
5. US Centers for Disease Control and Prevention. Summary of diagnostics among infants not passing hearing screening 2018. Available at: https://www.cdc.gov/ncbddd/hearingloss/2018-data/06-diagnostics.html.
6. Morton CC, Nance WE. Newborn hearing screening — A silent revolution. N Engl J Med 2006;354(20):2151–64.
7. Rudman J, Liu XZ. Genetics of hearing loss. Hearing J 2019;72(4):6–7.
8. Lieu JEC, Kenna M, Anne S, et al. Hearing loss in children: a review. JAMA 2020;324(21):2195–205.
9. Shearer AE, Shibata SB, Smith RJH. Genetic sensorineural hearing loss. In: Cummings otolaryngology - head and neck surgery vol. 150, 7th edition. Elsevier; 2021. p. 2279–92.
10. Inghamid NJ, Pearson SA, Vancollieid VE, et al. Mouse screen reveals multiple new genes underlying mouse and human hearing loss. PLoS Biol 2019;17(4):e3000194.

11. Shearer AE, Hildebrand MS, Smith RJ. Hereditary hearing loss and deafness overview. GeneReviews 1993;1–27.

12. Koffler T, Ushakov K, Avraham KB. Genetics of hearing loss: syndromic. Otolaryngol Clin North Am 2015;48(6):1041–61.

13. Wang Q, Xiang J, Sun J, et al. Nationwide population genetic screening improves outcomes of newborn screening for hearing loss in China. Genet Med 2019; 21(10):2231–8.

14. Azaiez H, Booth KT, Ephraim SS, et al. Genomic landscape and mutational signatures of deafness-associated genes. Am J Hum Genet 2018;103(4):484–97.

15. Hall WC, Smith SR, Sutter EJ, et al. Considering parental hearing status as a social determinant of deaf population health: insights from experiences of the "dinner table syndrome." PLoS One 2018;13(9):e0202169.

16. van Camp G, Smith R. Hereditary hearing loss - hereditary hearing loss homepage 2015. Available at: https://hereditaryhearingloss.org.

17. Chang KW. Genetics of hearing loss-nonsyndromic. Otolaryngol Clin North Am 2015;48(6):1063–72.

18. Sloan-Heggen CM, Bierer AO, Shearer AE, et al. Comprehensive genetic testing in the clinical evaluation of 1119 patients with hearing loss. Hum Genet 2016; 135(4):441–50.

19. Wang Q, Xue Y, Zhang Y, et al. Genetic basis of Y-linked hearing impairment. Am J Hum Genet 2013;92(2):301–6.

20. McDermott JH, Molina-Ramírez LP, Bruce IA, et al. Diagnosing and preventing hearing loss in the genomic age. Trends Hearing 2019;23:1–8.

21. McDermott JH, Mahood R, Stoddard D, et al. Pharmacogenetics to Avoid Loss of Hearing (PALOH) trial: a protocol for a prospective observational implementation trial. BMJ Open 2021;11(6):e044457.

22. Stark Z, Dolman L, Manolio TA, et al. Integrating genomics into healthcare: a global responsibility. Am J Hum Genet 2019;104(1):13–20.

23. Korver AMH, Smith RJH, van Camp G, et al. Congenital hearing loss. Nat Rev Dis Primers 2017;3:16094.

24. Boudewyns A, van den Ende J, Sommen M, et al. Role of targeted next generation sequencing in the etiological work-up of congenitally deaf children. Otol Neurotol 2018;39(6):732–8.

25. Boudewyns A, van den Ende J, Declau F, et al. Etiological work-up in referrals from neonatal hearing screening: 20 years of experience. Otology & neurotology 2020;41(9):1240–8.

26. Green GE, Scott DA, McDonald JM, et al. Performance of cochlear implant recipients with GJB2-related deafness. Am J Med Genet 2002;109(3):167–70.

27. Yan YJ, Li Y, Yang T, et al. The effect of GJB2 and SLC26A4 gene mutations on rehabilitative outcomes in pediatric cochlear implant patients. Eur Arch Otorhinolaryngol 2013;270(11):2865–70.

28. Shearer AE, Hansen MR. Auditory synaptopathy, auditory neuropathy, and cochlear implantation. Laryngoscope Invest Otolaryngol 2019;4(4):429–40.

29. Seligman KL, Shearer AE, Frees K, et al. Genetic causes of hearing loss in a large cohort of cochlear implant recipients. Otolaryngol Head Neck Surg 2021. https://doi.org/10.1177/01945998211021308. 019459982110213.

30. 2018 Summary of National CDC EHDI Data | Annual Data EHDI Program | CDC. Available at: https://www.cdc.gov/ncbddd/hearingloss/2018-data/01-data-summary.html. Accessed July 5, 2021.

31. Miller DT, Lee K, Chung WK, et al. ACMG SF v3.0 list for reporting of secondary findings in clinical exome and genome sequencing: a policy statement of the

American College of Medical Genetics and Genomics (ACMG). Genet Med 2021; 23(8):1381–90.

32. Dai P, Huang LH, Wang GJ, et al. Concurrent hearing and genetic screening of 180,469 neonates with follow-up in Beijing, China. Am J Hum Genet 2019; 105(4):803–12.

33. Wu CC, Tsai CH, Hung CC, et al. Newborn genetic screening for hearing impairment: a population-based longitudinal study. Genet Med 2017;19(1):6–12.

34. Minami SB, Mutai H, Nakano A, et al. GJB2-associated hearing loss undetected by hearing screening of newborns. Gene 2013;532(1):41–5.

35. Guo L, Xiang J, Sun L, et al. Concurrent hearing and genetic screening in a general newborn population. Hum Genet 2020;139(4):521–30.

36. Downie L, Halliday JL, Burt RA, et al. A protocol for whole-exome sequencing in newborns with congenital deafness: a prospective population-based cohort. BMJ Paediatr Open 2017;1(1):e000119.

37. Downie L, Halliday J, Lewis S, et al. Exome sequencing in newborns with congenital deafness as a model for genomic newborn screening: the Baby Beyond Hearing project. Genet Med 2020;22(5):937–44.

38. Downie L, Halliday J, Burt R, et al. Exome sequencing in infants with congenital hearing impairment: a population-based cohort study. Eur J Hum Genet 2020; 28(5):587–96.

39. Tutty E, Amor DJ, Halliday J, Lewis S, Martyn M, Goranitis I. Exome sequencing for isolated congenital hearing loss: a cost-effectiveness analysis. Laryngoscope 2021;131(7):E2371–7.

40. Downie L, Amor DJ, Halliday J, et al. Exome sequencing for isolated congenital hearing loss: a cost-effectiveness analysis. Laryngoscope 2020;131(7):E2371–7.

41. Khurana P, Cushing SL, Chakraborty PK, et al. Early hearing detection and intervention in Canada. Paediatr Child Health 2021;26(3):141–4.

42. Hearing loss risk factor screening. Newborn Screening Ontario. Available at: https://www.newbornscreening.on.ca/en/page/overview. Accessed June 24, 2021.

43. Pigeon BM, Gallagher LH, Dunn J. A World's first addition to Ontario's Infant Hearing Program. Canadian Audiologist; 2021;8(3):8–11.

44. Pfundt R, del Rosario M, Vissers LELM, et al. Detection of clinically relevant copy-number variants by exome sequencing in a large cohort of genetic disorders. Genet Med 2017;19(6):667–75.

45. Shearer AE, Kolbe DL, Azaiez H, et al. Copy number variants are a common cause of non-syndromic hearing loss. Genome Med 2014;6(5):37.

46. Peterson J, Nishimura C, Smith RJH. Genetic testing for congenital bilateral hearing loss in the context of targeted cytomegalovirus screening. Laryngoscope 2020;130(11):2714–8.

47. Raymond M, Walker E, Dave I, et al. Genetic testing for congenital non-syndromic sensorineural hearing loss. Int J Pediatr Otorhinolaryngol 2019;124:68–75.

48. Yoshinaga-Itano C, Sedey AL, Wiggin M, et al. Language outcomes improved through early hearing detection and earlier cochlear implantation. Otol Neurotol 2018;39(10):1256–63.

49. Nicolson T. Navigating hereditary hearing loss: pathology of the inner ear. Front Cell Neurosci 2021;15:1–7.

50. Schilder AGM, Su MP, Blackshaw H, et al. Hearing protection, restoration, and regeneration: an overview of emerging therapeutics for inner ear and central hearing disorders. Otol Neurotol 2019;40(5):559–70.

Auditory Neuropathy/ Auditory Synaptopathy

Linda J. Hood, PhD

KEYWORDS

- Auditory neuropathy • Auditory synaptopathy • Auditory evoked potentials
- Genetics

KEY POINTS

- Neural processing of auditory stimuli is affected in patients with auditory neuropathy/auditory synaptopathy (AN/AS).
- Physiologic measures, particularly auditory brainstem response and otoacoustic emissions, are needed to accurately identify AN/AS.
- Understanding of speech is poorer than expected, based on pure-tone threshold sensitivity.
- Patients vary widely in characteristics and management needs.

INTRODUCTION

The term auditory neuropathy (AN) was used by Starr and colleagues[1] to describe a group of patients who, unlike patients with typical sensorineural hearing loss (SNHL), demonstrated evidence of present cochlear (inner ear) activity that was accompanied by absent or highly abnormal neural responses at the level of the auditory nerve and brainstem. Several additional terms used to describe this hearing disorder include auditory neuropathy/dyssynchrony (AN/AD),[2] auditory neuropathy spectrum disorder (ANSD),[3] and auditory synaptopathy (AS).[4] Although these terms have associations with different underlying mechanisms or concepts, at present they often are used interchangeably. Future goals are to have accurate terminology that reflects underlying physiology; at present, the terms AN and AS are the closest to this goal. Thus, the term AN/AS will be used in this article. It should be understood that all terms (AN, AS, AN/AD, ANSD) will apply unless specifically noted. More accurate use of these and perhaps other descriptors will continue to emerge with advances in understanding of function and underlying processes.

Clinical presentation of patients with AN/AS typically indicates difficulty understanding speech, particularly in noisy situations. Although many patients with AN/AS demonstrate little or no ability to understand speech in quiet, some patients

Department of Hearing and Speech Sciences, Vanderbilt University Medical Center, 1215 21st Avenue South, Medical Center East, South Tower #8310, Nashville, TN 37232, USA
E-mail address: linda.j.hood@vanderbilt.edu

Otolaryngol Clin N Am 54 (2021) 1093–1100
https://doi.org/10.1016/j.otc.2021.07.004
0030-6665/21/© 2021 Elsevier Inc. All rights reserved.

oto.theclinics.com

demonstrate good word recognition ability, but only in quiet. All patients with AN/AS demonstrate difficulty listening in noisy situations with poorer word recognition ability than observed in persons with SNHL.[5] These factors can have significant impact on speech perception ability, and delayed speech and language development in infants and children is a common, although not universal, characteristic.

BACKGROUND

AN/AS is present in about 10% of individuals with auditory brainstem responses (ABR) that are either absent or highly abnormal as indicated by low-amplitude responses present only at high intensities, such as seen in patients with apparent severe or profound hearing loss. This estimate is based on data from several sources globally that include screening studies of infants and school-aged children.[6–9] A higher incidence of 17.3% and 15.4%, respectively, was reported among children identified with hearing loss following referral from newborn hearing screening.[10,11] Incidence in premature infants and among infants in the neonatal intensive care unit (NICU) is higher, with rates of AN/AS of 24% and higher.[12,13]

Clinical Audiologic Evaluation

Physiologic responses are key components in accurate identification and characterization of AN/AS (**Table 1**). Of the physiologic methods in present widespread clinical use, a combination of cochlear active process assays (otoacoustic emissions, OAE; cochlear microphonics, CM) and ABR forms the most sensitive combination of measures to assess AN/AS. In the absence of middle-ear disorders, OAEs are typically present in patients with AN/AS, although they might change over time in some patients. Because the CM is an electrical response, it is not dependent on reverse transmission back through the middle-ear system and, thus, might be observed in patients with middle-ear disorders where OAE recording is compromised. A key factor in distinguishing CM from a neural response is the reversal of the response with the change of the stimulus polarity from condensation to rarefaction polarity. The CM will invert, whereas neural responses typically do not completely invert.[14]

Table 1
Clinical characteristics and test results in patients with auditory neuropathy/auditory synaptopathy

Clinical Presentation
- Problems understanding speech in quiet and especially in noise, fluctuation, delayed speech/language development

Physiologic Measures	
Cochlear Active Processes	**Neural Responses**
• Present otoacoustic emissions (OAE) • Present cochlear microphonic (CM)	• Absent/abnormal auditory brainstem response (ABR) • Absent/abnormal middle-ear muscle reflex (MEMR) • Absent/abnormal medial olivocochlear reflex (MOCR)

Behavioral Measures
- Variable audiometric thresholds, configurations
- Generally poor, but variable speech recognition in quiet
- Poorer than expected speech recognition in noise

Neural responses from the eighth nerve/brainstem pathway are affected in these patients. ABRs are most often absent in patients with AN/AS, although some demonstrate evidence of limited, reduced neural synchrony for high-intensity signals. Berlin and colleagues[15] reported that approximately 75% of patients in their database had absent ABRs, whereas 25% showed abnormal responses characterized by the presence of low-amplitude Wave V only at high stimulus levels (typically in the range of 75–90 dB nHL [Average Hearing Level for brief stimuli in persons with normal hearing]). Evidence of interruption of neural function also is demonstrated by absent and/or abnormal efferent auditory reflexes: the middle ear muscle reflex[16] and the medial olivocochlear reflex.[17]

Behavioral responses, including pure-tone audiometry and speech recognition, are variable among patients with AN/AS. Pure-tone thresholds range from normal sensitivity to severe or profound hearing loss.[15,18] Threshold configurations vary and can be asymmetric between ears. In patients whose pure-tone thresholds exceed approximately 40 dB hearing level (HL) and OAEs are present, the disagreement between these 2 test results can provide a clue to the presence of AN/AS or another type of neural disorder that warrants further investigation.

Speech recognition is typically poorer with AN/AS than expected based on pure tone thresholds, but performance varies across individuals. Some patients demonstrate word recognition ability in quiet that is similar to persons with SNHL, whereas word recognition ability in noise for AN/AS patients is below what is expected in SNHL.[1,5,19] In a group of patients aged 4 years and older where word recognition was measured using standardized tests, Berlin and colleagues[15] reported that 56% of the patients had no measurable word recognition ability, even in quiet. The remaining patients had word recognition scores in quiet that varied from poor to excellent.[15,20] In contrast, it is important to note that only 7% of the patients in this cohort had measurable word recognition in noise, and scores for all were poorer than observed in SNHL.[5,15] The variable, and generally poor, speech recognition ability presents a particular challenge in planning appropriate management.

Underlying Mechanisms

The clinical test results observed in patients with AN/AS can occur as a result of the absence or disruption of inner hair cell (IHC) activity, interruption in function of the synapse of the IHC and auditory nerve, and/or abnormalities of the auditory nerve. Gene mutations associated with AN have been identified, with variable inheritance patterns. AN/AS is seen in nonsyndromic recessive inheritance, as well as part of a syndrome, such as hereditary motor sensory neuropathies. AN/AS can be distinguished as presynaptic or postsynaptic in origin, based on physiologic response characteristics and underlying genetics.[4,21–24] An example of a synaptic form (AS) involves the OTOF gene that encodes otoferlin, a protein that plays a crucial role in the function of the IHC ribbon synapses.[25,26] Postsynaptic forms of AN include patients with hereditary motor-sensory neuropathies, such as Charcot-Marie-Tooth disease and Friedreich ataxia.[22]

Variation Among Patients with Auditory Neuropathy/Auditory Synaptopathy

Some patients with AN/AS demonstrate fluctuation in hearing over time. In a limited number of cases, fluctuation in hearing has been linked to changes in body temperature.[27,28] Most AN/AS patients show bilateral characteristics, although function can be asymmetric between ears, and cases of unilateral AN/AS have been documented. Some patients have risk factors, and some forms are accompanied by neural problems in other systems. It should be noted that many patients with AN/AS have no risk factors and no evidence of abnormal function other than hearing loss.

Auditory Neuropathy/Auditory Synaptopathy in Infants

Infants at risk for AN/AS are identified at birth in newborn hearing screening programs that use ABR as the screening tool. Programs that use OAEs as the screening tool will miss these infants, resulting in late identification, often when parental concern about speech and language delay arises. The Joint Committee on Infant Hearing[29] recommends ABR testing for infants in the NICU based on the higher risk for AN/AS in the NICU population. Infants with present OAEs and poor or absent ABR are considered "at risk" because the ABR continues to mature through the first 12 to 18 months after birth. Some infants who show AN/AS characteristics at birth develop an ABR over the first year of life; however, the number of these infants is low.[30,31] It is important to monitor infants suspected of having AN/AS closely over at least the first year of life with appropriate, sensitive measures.

Management Approaches and Outcomes

Variation in underlying mechanisms and variable clinical characteristics among patients dictate the need for individual management approaches. Modifications in management might be needed, particularly in cases whereby auditory function changes over time. Because discrimination of sound generally is affected to a much greater degree than detection of sound, decision making and management planning should consider clarity of sound and suprathreshold function.

Amplification

Trial of amplification is recommended, although variation in benefit among patients should be anticipated. A key component of benefit involves improved sound discrimination, which is necessary to facilitate speech and language development and support auditory communication. Studies report variable benefit from hearing aids, even with appropriately audible signals (eg, Refs.[15,32]). When assessing benefit and making decisions related to proceeding from amplification to cochlear implantation, it is important to separate ability to detect sound from ability to discriminate sound. If a child is not progressing, particularly after several months of hearing aid use, then cochlear implantation may be recommended for a patient and family to consider.[31]

Assistive listening systems

Patients typically benefit from use of assistive listening systems, such as remote microphone technology (alone or with other devices), consistent with the particular difficulty that AN/AS patients experience in noisy situations.[33] When clear auditory information is not accessible, then inclusion of visual information will facilitate language development in infants and children and assist in difficult listening situations.[34]

Cochlear implants

Children and adults demonstrate improved speech perception ability and speech and language development with cochlear implants.[15,35] Importantly, cochlear implants have been shown to facilitate perception of speech in quiet and in noise, and synchronous neural responses are observed on ABRs and other physiologic measures using electrical stimuli. Outcomes with cochlear implants have been studied in patients with genetically defined presynaptic and postsynaptic forms of AN/AS. Santarelli and colleagues[23] demonstrated success with cochlear implants in patients with AS associated with OTOF mutations. A postsynaptic form of AN associated with certain mutations in the OPA1 gene showed good, although variable, outcomes with cochlear implants.[24]

DISCUSSION: THE FUTURE

Discovery will continue to promote understanding of AN/AS and facilitate accurate diagnosis and effective management. As noted previously, advances in both diagnostic assays of auditory function and genetic analysis will facilitate the ability to differentiate disrupted auditory nerve activity (AN), synaptic activity (AS), disordered IHC function, and accurately define genotype-phenotype relationships.

The development of sensitive methods to evaluate auditory function that can be implemented in clinical settings has the potential to move the field forward in clarifying individual characteristics and linking results to specific underlying mechanisms. Cortical auditory evoked potentials, present in many AN/AS patients, show promise as an objective method to evaluate sound detection, as it is not possible with ABR (eg, Refs.[36,37]). Importantly, studies linking cortical response presence and speech perception ability are promising in the evaluation of patients with AN/AS who cannot provide reliable behavioral responses.[38–40]

Accurate differential diagnosis, particularly among conditions that have similar patient presentation, such as cochlear nerve deficiency, enlarged vestibular aqueduct, and centrally based auditory processing, will be helpful in understanding sources of variation. Following patients over time will provide important information to understand the natural history of various forms of AN/AS, and identification of factors that contribute to fluctuation and progression.

SUMMARY

Advances in characterizing underlying mechanisms, identifying genetic mutations associated with AN/AS, and sensitively assaying auditory function will promote accurate evaluation and management of patients with AN/AS. Progress will include the development and clinical implementation of methods that can accurately distinguish normal from abnormal function at IHC, synaptic, and neural levels, the identification of specific factors related to various types of AN/AS, and connections between characteristics and outcomes. Advances will have a positive impact on management and provide knowledge to guide patients and their families in making informed decisions.

CLINICS CARE POINTS

- Auditory neuropathy/auditory synaptopathy is associated with compromised neural processing of auditory stimuli.
  - Detection of sound is inconsistent with speech understanding, particularly for listening to speech in noise.
- Assessment of auditory function using physiologic measures, which include the auditory brainstem response and otoacoustic emissions, is needed to accurately identify patients with auditory neuropathy/auditory synaptopathy.
- Genetic evaluation can provide information about underlying mechanisms and inform management.
- Progress related to intervention should be monitored with formal evaluation and at regular intervals.
  - For infants and children, with measures of speech and language development.
  - For children and adults, with speech perception testing, including testing in noise.
- Patients vary widely in characteristics and management needs.
  - Follow patients closely and consider the possibility of change over time.

DISCLOSURE

Research supported by the National Institutes of Health, National Institute on Deafness and Other Communication Disorders (NIH-NIDCD). Consultant for Akouos, Inc and Pfizer, Inc. There are no conflicts with the content of this material.

REFERENCES

1. Starr A, Picton TW, Sininger Y, et al. Auditory neuropathy. Brain 1996;119:741–53.
2. Berlin C, Hood L, Rose K. On renaming auditory neuropathy as auditory dys-synchrony: implications for a clearer understanding of the underlying mechanisms and management options. Audiol Today 2001;13:15–7.
3. Hayes D, Sininger Y, editor. Guidelines Development Conference on the Identification and Management of Infants with Auditory Neuropathy. Como (Italy): 2008.
4. Moser T, Starr A. Auditory neuropathy – neural and synaptic mechanisms. Nat Rev Neurol 2016;12:135–49.
5. Rance G, Barker E, Mok M, et al. Speech perception in noise for children with auditory neuropathy/dys-synchrony type hearing loss. Ear Hear 2007;28:351–60.
6. Berlin CI, Hood LJ, Morlet T, et al. The search for auditory neuropathy patients and connexin 26 patients in schools for the deaf. ARO Abstr 2000;23:23.
7. Lee JSM, McPherson B, Yuen KCP, et al. Screening for auditory neuropathy in a school for hearing impaired children. Int J Pediatr Otolaryngol 2001;61:39–46.
8. Rance G, Beer DE, Cone-Wesson B, et al. Clinical findings for a group of infants and young children with auditory neuropathy. Ear Hear 1999;20:238–52.
9. Sininger YS. Auditory neuropathy in infants and children: implications for early hearing detection and intervention programs. Audiol Today 2000;14:16–21.
10. Kirkim G, Serbetcioglu B, Erdag TK, et al. The frequency of auditory neuropathy detected by universal newborn hearing screening program. Int J Pediatr Otorhinolaryngol 2008;72:1461–9.
11. Ngo RYS, Tan HKK, Balakrishnan A, et al. Auditory neuropathy/auditory dys-synchrony detected by universal newborn hearing screening. Int J Pediatr Otorhinolaryngol 2006;70:1299–306.
12. Berg AL, Spitzer SB, Towers HM, et al. Newborn hearing screening in the NICU: profile of failed auditory brainstem response/passed otoacoustic emission. Pediatrics 2005;116:933–8.
13. Rea PA, Gibson WPR. Evidence for surviving outer hair cell function in congenitally deaf ears. Laryngoscope 2003;113:2030–4.
14. Berlin CI, Bordelon J, John P St, et al. Reversing click polarity may uncover auditory neuropathy in infants. Ear Hear 1998;19:37–47.
15. Berlin CI, Hood LJ, Morlet T, et al. Multi-site diagnosis and management of 260 patients with auditory neuropathy/dys-synchrony (auditory neuropathy spectrum disorder). Int J Audiol 2010;49:30–43.
16. Berlin CI, Hood LJ, Morlet T, et al. Absent or elevated middle ear muscle reflexes in the presence of normal otoacoustic emissions: a universal finding in 136 cases of auditory neuropathy/dys-synchrony. J Am Acad Audiol 2005;16:546–53.
17. Hood LJ, Berlin CI, Bordelon J, et al. Patients with auditory neuropathy/dys-synchrony lack efferent suppression of transient evoked otoacoustic emissions. J Am Acad Audiol 2003;14:302–13.
18. Kaga K, Nakamura M, Shinogami M, et al. Auditory nerve disease of both ears revealed by auditory brainstem responses, electrocochleography and otoacoustic emissions. Scand Audiol 1996;25:233–8.

19. Zeng FG, Oba S, Garde S, et al. Temporal and speech processing deficits in auditory neuropathy. Neuroreport 1999;10:3429–35.
20. Yellin MW, Jerger J, Fifer RC. Norms for disproportionate loss in speech intelligibility. Ear Hear 1989;10:231–4.
21. McMahon CM, Patuzzi RB, Gibson WPR, et al. Frequency-specific electrococochleography indicates that presynaptic and postsynaptic mechanisms of auditory neuropathy exist. Ear Hear 2008;29:314–25.
22. Rance G, Starr A. Pathophysiological mechanisms and functional hearing consequences of auditory neuropathy. Brain 2015;138:3141–58.
23. Santarelli R, del Castillo I, Cama E, et al. Audibility, speech perception and processing of temporal cues in ribbon synaptic disorders due to OTOF mutations. Hear Res 2015;330:200–12.
24. Santarelli R, Rossi R, Scimemi P, et al. OPA1-related auditory neuropathy: site of lesion and outcome of cochlear implantation. Brain 2015;138:563–76.
25. Rodríguez-Ballesteros M, Reynoso R, Olarte M, et al. A multicenter study on the prevalence and spectrum of mutations in the otoferlin gene (OTOF) in subjects with nonsyndromic hearing impairment and auditory neuropathy. Hum Mut 2008;29:823–31.
26. Varga R, Kelley PM, Keats BJ, et al. Non-syndromic recessive auditory neuropathy is the results of mutations in the otoferlin (OTOF) gene. J Med Genet 2003;40: 45–50.
27. Marlin S, Feldmann D, Nguyen Y, et al. Temperature-sensitive auditory neuropathy associated with an otoferlin mutation: deafening fever! Biochem Biophys Res Comm 2010;394:737–42.
28. Starr A, Sininger Y, Winter M, et al. Transient deafness due to temperature-sensitive auditory neuropathy. Ear Hear 1998;19:169–79.
29. Joint Committee on Infant Hearing. Year 2019 position statement: principles and guidelines for early hearing detection and intervention programs. J Early Hear Detect Interv 2019;4:1–44.
30. Attias J, Raveh E. Transient deafness in young candidates for cochlear implants. Audiol Neurotol 2007;12:325–33.
31. Hayes C, Watkins L, Edwards M, et al. Auditory neuropathy/auditory dys-synchrony. Nashville (TN): Poster presentation 2010;TAASLP.
32. Roush P, Frymark T, Venediktov R, et al. Audiologic management of auditory neuropathy spectrum disorder in children: a systematic review of the literature. Am J Audiol 2011;20:159–70.
33. Hood LJ, Wilensky D, Li L, et al. The role of FM technology in the management of patients with auditory neuropathy/dys-synchrony. Proc Internat Conf FM Technol 2004; Chicago, Illinois.
34. Berlin CI, Li L, Hood LJ, et al. Auditory neuropathy/dys-synchrony: after the diagnosis, then what? Sem Hear 2002;23:209–14.
35. Breneman AI, Gifford RH, Dejong MD. Cochlear implantation in children with auditory neuropathy spectrum disorder: long-term outcomes. J Am Acad Audiol 2012;23:5–17.
36. Gardner-Berry K, Purdy SC, TYC Ching, et al. The audiological journey and early outcomes of twelve infants with auditory neuropathy spectrum disorder from birth to two years of age. Int J Audiol 2015;54:524–35.
37. He S, Grose JH, Teagle HF, et al. Acoustically evoked auditory change complex in children with auditory neuropathy spectrum disorder: a potential objective tool for identifying cochlear implant candidates. Ear Hear 2015;36:289–301.

38. Narne VK, Vanaja CS. Speech identification and cortical potentials in individuals with auditory neuropathy. Behav Brain Funct 2008;31:4–15.
39. Pearce W, Golding M, Dillon H. Cortical auditory evoked potentials in the assessment of auditory neuropathy: two cases. J Am Acad Audiol 2007;18:380–90.
40. Rance G, Cone-Wesson B, Wunderlich J, et al. Speech perception and cortical event related potentials in children with auditory neuropathy. Ear Hear 2002;23:239–53.

Mechanisms of Ototoxicity and Otoprotection

Peter S. Steyger, PhD

KEYWORDS

- Cochleotoxicity • Vestibulotoxicity • Aminoglycosides
- Platinum-based therapeutics • Blood-labyrinth barrier • Ototoxicity monitoring
- Ototherapeutics

KEY POINTS

- Numerous hospital-prescribed medications and environmental factors cause ototoxicity.
- Ototoxicity encompasses hearing loss (cochleotoxicity) and/or balance deficits (vestibulotoxicity).
- Ototoxicity has permanent, lifelong debilitating consequences, and if uncorrected it can lead to unfulfilled scholastic and career trajectories in children, as well as accelerated cognitive decline in aging individuals.
- Otoprotection to preserve or restore auditory and/or vestibular function includes ototoxicity monitoring, prosthetic and social rehabilitation, and soon, pharmaceutical ototherapeutics to preserve, repair, or restore inner ear functions.
- Ototoxicity is, ideally, a preventable form of acquired hearing loss or vestibular deficit.

SIGNIFICANCE

The Ototoxicity Working Group of Pharmaceutical Interventions for Hearing Loss defined ototoxicity as damage to the inner ear, targeting cochlear and vestibular structures as well as sensory function, due to exposure to certain pharmaceuticals, chemicals, and/or ionizing radiation. Ototoxicity typically focuses on the inner ear; however, ototoxins can also affect central auditory pathways and are, thus, considered neurotoxic.[1,2] Ototoxins can also cause kidney damage and associated renal dysfunction.[3–5] This review focuses primarily on ototoxic hospital-based medications received by several hundred thousand infants and children in Western Europe and the Americas each year—aminoglycoside antibiotics and the anticancer drug, cisplatin. Other clinically-relevant drugs are listed in **Table 1**.

Aminoglycoside antibiotics, like gentamicin, are clinically-relevant, broad-spectrum medications to treat life-threatening bacterial infections, often of unknown cause,

Translational Hearing Center, Biomedical Sciences, Creighton University, 2500 California Plaza, Omaha, NE 68178, USA
E-mail address: petersteyger@creighton.edu

oto.theclinics.com

Table 1
Major classes of ototoxic drugs (with specific examples)

Class	Examples
Platinum-based therapeutics	Cisplatin, carboplatin, oxaliplatin
Aminoglycosides	Amikacin, gentamicin, tobramycin
Peptide antibiotics	Capreomycin, viomycin, chloramphenicol
Polypeptide antibiotics	Vancomycin (and synergistic with aminoglycosides)
Macrolides	Erythromycin
Cyclodextrins (vehicle)	Derivatives of cyclodextrins, eg, for Niemann-Pick syndrome type 1C
Antimalarials	Chloroquine, hydrochloroquine
Antirheumatics	Chloroquine, hydrochloroquine
Loop diuretics	Furosemide, bumetanide (and synergistic with aminoglycosides or cisplatin)
Nonsteroidal anti-inflammatory drugs	Acetaminophen (a.k.a. paracetamol)
Antineoplastics	Vincristine

Adapted from Steyger PS. Mechanisms of Aminoglycoside- and Cisplatin-induced Ototoxicity. American Journal of Audiology. 2021;in press, with permission from Cold Spring Harbor Press.

including neonatal sepsis, mycobacterial infections, and meningitis. Exacerbated respiratory infections in children with cystic fibrosis are typically treated with tobramycin or amikacin, and individuals, with tuberculosis with kanamycin, and these are also aminoglycoside antibiotics. Aminoglycoside-induced hearing loss is typically cumulatively dose dependent,[6,7] and the incidence in humans is as high as 20% to 63% of those receiving multiday dosing.[7–11] The prevalence of aminoglycoside-induced vestibular deficits is underreported because of the widespread lack of clinical instrumentation for assessing vestibular function.[12]

Liver tumors and glioblastomas in the brains of children are effectively diminished by cisplatin or other platinum-based derivatives like carboplatin and oxaliplatin, and the degree of drug-induced hearing loss is typically dose dependent.[13–15] There are fewer reports of cisplatin-induced vestibular deficits in children owing to the lack of routine clinical assessments,[12,16] although there are preclinical reports of dose-dependent cisplatin-induced vestibular deficits.[17] Children with Niemann-Pick type 1C syndrome can be treated with derivatives of cyclodextrins, a primary component of drug formulations, which at higher doses also sequester membrane cholesterols.[18] Treatment with these pharmacologic agents in clinical settings can cause ototoxicity. Environmental ototoxins include solvents[19–21] and metals (eg, lead, copper).[22–25]

Uncorrected congenital or acquired hearing loss in infants and children can lead to delayed acquisition of listening and spoken language skills compared with age-matched peers with typical hearing, with concomitant delays in achieving academic, linguistic, and psychosocial milestones.[26,27] Loss of vestibular function is also debilitating.[28,29] There is an estimated socioeconomic cost greater than $1.5 million over the lifetime of each prelingually deafened child (in 2019 dollars).[30]

CROSSING THE BLOOD-LABYRINTH BARRIER

The inner ear is protected by a blood-labyrinth barrier (BLB, akin to the blood-brain barrier) that compartmentalizes inner ear cells and fluids from the bloodstream and the rest of the body. Endothelial cells lining the cochlear blood vessels are coupled together by tight junctions to prevent extravasation (ie, the paracellular trafficking of blood cells, macromolecules, and serum from the capillary into cochlear tissues).[31] Within the cochlea, there are 2 major fluid spaces, perilymph and endolymph. Blood-borne ototoxins are readily trafficked into the perilymph surrounding the basolateral membranes of hair cells,[32,33] yet this does not seem to be the primary entry route into hair cells[34] (**Fig. 1**). Instead, aminoglycosides and cisplatin cross the BLB of the stria vascularis and, from there, appear to be rapidly cleared into endolymph and enter hair cells across their apical membranes more readily than when directly infused into the perilymph.[34–37] The cellular and molecular mechanisms by which aminoglycosides and cisplatin cross the BLB and transverse the tight-junction-coupled marginal cells of the stria vascularis into endolymph remain to be determined and likely include one or more of the following molecular mechanisms: ion channels, transporters, exchangers, or transcytosis,[12,38] each permutation specific for each individual class of ototoxins.

ENTRY OF OTOTOXINS INTO SENSORY HAIR CELLS

Typically, cochleotoxicity requires ototoxins to enter hair cells.[39] At the distal tips of most stereocilia in the mechanically-sensitive hair bundle are transduction channels (**Fig. 2**A) that allow the polycationic aminoglycosides to permeate into the cell.[40] These transduction channels are nonselective cation channels such as TMC1.[41] Aminoglycoside permeation of TMC1 channels can be blocked by polyvalent cations like magnesium or calcium (**Fig. 2**B), as well as by organic compounds like curare and quinine.[42,43] Hair cells also express other aminoglycoside-permeant channels, including several transient receptor potential (TRP) channels, each activated by different physical or chemical stimuli[44]; these include TRPV1 and TRPV4 at the apical membrane of hair cells (**Fig. 2**C).[45–48] The aminoglycoside-permeant TRPA1 channel is likely expressed on the basolateral membranes of outer hair cells (**Fig. 2**D).[49]

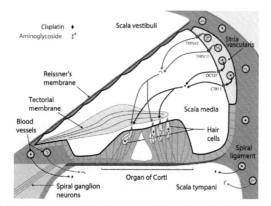

Fig. 1. Primary trafficking routes of aminoglycosides and cisplatin from the vasculature to cochlear hair cells. Circulating ototoxins typically enter the cochlea via capillaries in the stria vascularis and are cleared into endolymph via as-yet-unidentified ion channels or transporters, although several candidates exist, for example, TRPV1 and TRPV4 nonselective cation channels for aminoglycosides, and potentially via OCT2 and CTR1 transporters for cisplatin. Once in endolymph, the ototoxins can enter the hair cells via one or more of several mechanisms. (*From* Kros CJ, Steyger PS. Aminoglycoside- and Cisplatin-Induced Ototoxicity: Mechanisms and Otoprotective Strategies. Cold Spring Harb Perspect Med. 2019;9(11), with permission from Cold Spring Harbor Press.)

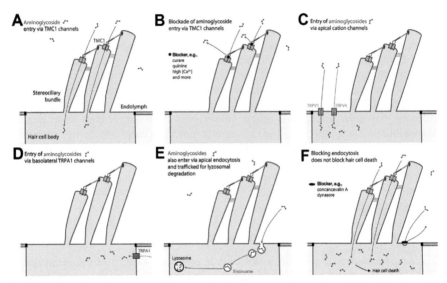

Fig. 2. Aminoglycoside entry into hair cells. Aminoglycosides preferentially enter mammalian hair cells via the TMC1 channel that consists of 2 TMC subunits (*purple*), each with a permeation groove (*A*). Entry of aminoglycosides can be blocked by curare, quinine, and high levels of polyvalent cations (*B*). Other aminoglycoside-permeant channels on the apical membrane of hair cells include TRPV1 and TPRV4 (*C*), and TRPA1 on the basolateral membrane of outer hair cells (*D*). (*E*) Nonspecific endocytosis enables aminoglycoside-laden endosomes to traffic to hair cell lysosomes. (*F*) Blocking endocytosis does not prevent hair cell death when aminoglycosides can enter hair cells via the TMC1 channel. (*From* Steyger PS. Mechanisms of Aminoglycoside- and Cisplatin-induced Ototoxicity. American Journal of Audiology. 2021;in press, with permission from the American Journal of Audiology.)

Aminoglycosides can also enter hair cells via nonreceptor-mediated endocytosis and are trafficked to lysosomes (**Fig. 2**E). Blocking endocytosis (**Fig. 2**F) or impeding intracellular trafficking of aminoglycoside-laden endosomes does not prevent hair cell death.[42,50,51] Cisplatin can enter cells via passive diffusion across the cell membrane (**Fig. 3**A).[52] Hair cells with active (open) transduction channels (**Fig. 3**B) are more susceptible to cisplatin-induced cytotoxicity.[53]

Once in cochlear hair cells, cochleotoxic dosing with aminoglycosides and cisplatin first leads to outer hair cell death in the basal high-frequency region of the cochlea, particularly in outer hair cells. Increasing cumulative dosing leads to further outer hair cell death in more apical regions of the cochlea (ie, at lower frequencies) and inner hair cell death, with an increasing risk of permanent hearing loss.[7,15,54] There is one major difference between aminoglycosides and cisplatin, and that is the preferential cochleotoxicity of cisplatin, compared with the more equal reporting of cochleotoxicity and vestibulotoxicity induced by aminoglycosides, although the underlying cause for this difference remains hypothetical.[55]

There are multiple (yet incompletely defined) molecular mechanisms of hair cell death, and the best characterizations for aminoglycosides and cisplatin are reviewed elsewhere.[4,5,12] It is important to stress that ototoxicity does not depend on hair cell dysfunction or cell death and can dysregulate nonsensory cells within the inner ear essential for sensitive auditory perception (eg, the stria vascularis).[12] In the following section, we focus on the clinical settings that can exacerbate the degree of hearing loss and vestibular disorders induced by ototoxins, particularly by aminoglycosides and cisplatin.

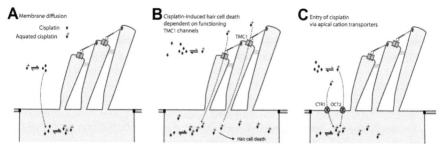

Fig. 3. Cisplatin entry into hair cells. (A) Cisplatin has multiple potential entry routes. Neutral cisplatin can diffuse across the plasma membrane and is readily aquated in the cytoplasm to the more toxic form of cisplatin that can form functionally disruptive adducts with proteins and DNA. (B) Uptake of aquated cisplatin depends on functional TMC channel complexes. (C) Cellular uptake of the aquated form of cisplatin can also occur via CTR1 and OCT2 transport proteins when expressed by the cell. (*From* Steyger PS. Mechanisms of Aminoglycoside- and Cisplatin-induced Ototoxicity. American Journal of Audiology. 2021;in press, with permission from the American Journal of Audiology.)

CLINICAL SETTINGS THAT CAN EXACERBATE THE RISK OF DRUG-INDUCED HEARING LOSS

Experimentally induced inflammation (to mimic host-mounted responses to bacterial infection) exacerbates the degree of aminoglycoside- and cisplatin-induced hearing loss in mice,[38,48,56] and potentially for vestibulotoxicity.[57] Pilot studies of neonates treated with aminoglycosides likely confirm these preclinical findings.[58,59] Aminoglycoside-induced lysis of bacteria elevates the inflammatory response (ie, the Jarisch-Herxheimer reaction).[60,61] The mechanisms underlying the potentiation of hearing loss by inflammation remain to be established.[62,63] Thus, the very patients with bacterial infections (and therefore inflammation) treated with aminoglycosides are likely at higher risk of ototoxin-induced hearing loss.[38]

Other clinical settings can also exacerbate the risk of drug-induced hearing loss and include renal insufficiency decreasing the clearance of ototoxins from blood,[64,65] increasing age with concomitant decreased glomerular filtration rate,[66–69] depletion of endogenous antioxidants needed to ameliorate ototoxin-induced generation of toxic levels of reactive oxygen species,[70–72] fever (hyperthermia or higher-than-normal body temperature),[59,73] and transient ischemia/hypoxia.[74] Aminoglycoside- and cisplatin-induced cochleotoxicity is also greater when these ototoxins are administered during active hours (ie, nighttime for rodents).[75–78]

Several single nucleotide polymorphisms in mitochondrial ribosomal RNA (eg, A1555G and C1494T) result in a higher binding affinity to aminoglycosides, leading to mistranslation of mRNA and inaccurate protein synthesis and a greater susceptibility to aminoglycoside-induced hearing loss.[79–82] At this time, no genomic polymorphisms have been reported to modulate susceptibility to aminoglycoside-induced hearing loss. Several genomic polymorphisms have been reported to increase the risk of cisplatin-induced hearing loss, including gene variants for antioxidant enzymes, DNA adduct repair enzymes, antioxidant enzymes, drug efflux, or membrane pumps.[83–86] However, the predictive value of these genomic variants in predisposing individuals for drug-induced ototoxicity is currently poor.[87,88]

Hospitalized children frequently receive multiple medications simultaneously, and several clinically-relevant nonototoxic drugs can potentiate drug-induced hearing loss. For example, the neuromuscular blocking agent pancuronium bromide is frequently prescribed for neonates requiring respiratory assistance (via intubation and ventilation); however, pancuronium bromide can potentiate the cochleotoxicity of loop diuretics prescribed for hypervolemic patients.[89,90] Simultaneous dosing with 2 or more ototoxic therapeutics can synergistically exacerbate the degree of ototoxicity to greater than the sum of the 2 ototoxins alone. These cotherapeutics include aminoglycosides and loop diuretics in hypertensive individuals,[91–93] or aminoglycosides with vancomycin, a glycopeptide antibiotic commonly prescribed in the neonatal intensive care unit.[94,95] Enhanced ototoxicity can also occur when cisplatin is coadministered with aminoglycosides, loop diuretics, and cranial radiation.[96–99] Thus, when dosing with multiple drugs simultaneously, all therapeutics should be examined for toxic interactions, including potentiated or synergistic ototoxic effects, and alternative dosing regimens identified where possible.

Loud sound exposures exacerbate the degree of aminoglycoside-induced ototoxicity.[100–102] Noise exposure also increases cisplatin-induced hearing loss.[103–106] These data are relevant when children require pharmacotherapy following recent exposure to intense loud sounds.

OTOPROTECTION

Strategies that protect the inner ear from the toxic effects of ototoxins in children are currently considered to be the same as those being developed for adults. Multiple strategies have been investigated, although few have completed phase 3 clinical trials and none are yet approved by the US Food and Drug Administration (FDA) in the United States. The most intensely investigated strategy to prevent ototoxicity has been efforts to inhibit the toxic generation of reactive oxygen/nitrogen species or the production of proapoptotic factors.[15,107,108] Potentially more specific, otoprotective strategies now include blocking systemically administered ototoxins from crossing the BLB and entering the inner ear fluids to prevent toxicity,[12] and physicochemical structural modification of ototoxins to prevent entry into hair cells and thus ameliorate ototoxicity while retaining their desired therapeutic efficacy has also been investigated,[109,110] although for derivatives of cisplatin, this has led to reduced clinical efficacy (ie, toxicity to the tumor) despite decreased ototoxicity.[15]

Alternative delivery strategies have focused on local delivery to the middle or inner ear to reduce the systemic toxicity associated with oral or parenteral administration of candidate otoprotective compounds; however, local delivery has challenges too, principally rapid clearance from the middle or inner ear.[111] One strategy to reduce clearance has been to use hydrogels and nanoparticles to retain the drug in the vicinity of the round window membrane. One novel strategy is to inject drug-loaded magnetic nanoparticles onto the round window and use a contralateral magnet to pull the magnetic nanoparticles into the inner ear. This strategy abrogated cisplatin-induced hearing loss in the high-frequency (basal) region of the cochlea.[112]

Unbiased Screening

Many of the aforementioned strategies to prevent ototoxicity used a rational, deductive approach to selecting and designing otoprotective dosing regimens and have been clearly successful preclinically to varying degrees. An alternative strategy has emerged in recent years to use unbiased screening of large compound libraries in silico, in vitro, and/or using zebrafish larvae to identify promising ototoxic "hits" or candidate otoprotective compounds.

Computational, or in vitro, models use molecular structures and physiochemical properties to predict drug toxicity or efficacy in an unbiased manner, based on reported structure-activity relationships. This approach has been used to predict cardio- or hepatotoxicity.[113,114] Two studies have reported in silico screening strategies for ototoxicity, whereas others use pathway or linkage models (https://lincsproject.org/LINCS) to identify potential otoprotectants.[62,115] Promising hits or candidate otoprotective compounds identified in silico must be verified using in vitro or in vivo assays. In vitro assays typically use cell lines, including those derived from the cochlea.[116–118] Although cell lines do not possess stereocilia with mechanically gated TMC1 channels, cell lines are extremely useful for deciphering the molecular and signaling pathways underlying ototoxic or otoprotective mechanisms.[118–121]

Like most fish, zebrafish possess on the surface of their body a mechanosensitive lateral line consisting of neuromasts within which are sensory hair cells with stereocilia and mechanically gated transduction channels, analogous to cochlear and vestibular hair cells. Female zebrafish release hundreds of larvae in each clutch, and within 4 to 5 days after fertilization they have functional neuromasts.[122] These numbers and ease of access (without a BLB) enable medium-throughput screening of compound libraries to identify hits that induce hair cell toxicity,[62] or interact with hair cell transduction channels to protect neuromast hair cells from aminoglycoside or cisplatin cytotoxicity.[123–125] Subsequently, these hits or candidate otoprotective compounds need to be validated preclinically using inner ear explants and in vivo ototoxicity models, primarily rodents and higher-order mammals, before advancing to human clinical trials.[117,118,124]

CHALLENGES TO PREVENTING OTOTOXICITY

We do not yet appreciate the numerous ways each ototoxin can induce cytotoxicity; this is best exemplified by the hundreds of observed aminoglycoside- or cisplatin-binding proteins, most of which remain unidentified and therefore uncharacterized, of which a fraction will have cytotoxic interactions and the remainder incidental, benign, or even cytoprotective interactions.[120,121,126] Hair cells and strial cells (like renal proximal tubule cells) are often unable to clear ototoxins from their cytosol.[35,127] Most other cells within the body are typically able to clear ototoxins from their cytosol, often by as-yet-unknown mechanisms; the reasons for these differences in toxicologic sensitivities remain highly speculative.

If candidate otoprotective compounds are to be delivered orally or systemically, and the primary site of otoprotection is within the inner ear itself, these compounds must first cross the BLB at sufficient quantities to meet therapeutic levels without being systemically toxic. If this is not possible, local delivery via intratympanic administration might be viable if the candidate otoprotective compounds are efficacious in the perilymph. Other crucial research-driven questions have been posed elsewhere.[102]

Although knowledge of the mechanism by which therapeutic compounds achieve their efficacy is not always needed for FDA approval, the mechanisms by which candidate compounds provide their otoprotective effect are increasingly being requested, and can add years to the discovery pipeline before a drug can be advanced to clinical trials. This phenomenon can be abrogated by repurposing already FDA-approved drugs for other indications to off-label indications if otoprotection can be shown preclinically (eg, statins).[128,129] Candidate otoprotective compounds must be effective in the medical settings in which they will be used (eg, in individuals with host-mounted inflammatory responses to infection or cancer treatment [eg, radiation]). This practice has been robustly implemented for pharmaceutical interventions for loud sound exposures, but not for prevention of ototoxicity in sick individuals.

Several nonpharmacologic, yet otoprotective or rehabilitative interventions, are also likely in the near future. The identification of risk factors, including aging, renal insufficiency, inflammation, genetic polymorphisms, or selected cotherapeutics, that predispose individuals to a greater risk of ototoxicity can be extracted from the medical record or tested for. For example, clinical guidelines exist for identifying which currently known mitochondrial polymorphisms predispose individuals to ototoxicity.[82] In such cases, nonototoxic pharmacotherapies can be prescribed. Even if these alternate routes can be more expensive in the short-term, they would still be much cheaper than the socioeconomic costs over the individual's lifetime. Additional nonpharmacologic otoprotective strategies include developing point-of-care (bedside) diagnostic procedures for sepsis through species-specific detection of microbial DNA sequences[130] or genomic screening for genomic polymorphisms that enhance susceptibility to drug-induced ototoxicity.[86,131]

Nonetheless, at present, the prevalence and incidence of most predisposing factors remain uncertain due to the variability of each subject's medical and ototoxin dosing history within a population. Given the need to prescribe ototoxic medications to individuals in life-threatening situations, it is important to implement ototoxicity monitoring protocols as recommended for those with cystic fibrosis.[132] Widespread implementation of ototoxicity monitoring protocols will provide new insights into the prevalence and incidence of cochleotoxicity and vestibulotoxicity that will accelerate the relative significance and impact of ototoxicity on quality-of-life scores and optimal rehabilitation of those affected by drug-induced hearing loss.

CLINICS CARE POINTS

- The degree of expected ototoxicity from multiday dosing with known ototoxins can be amplified by risk factors such as renal insufficiency or systemic inflammation.
- Dosing with multiple pharmacotherapeutics simultaneously (even if separated temporally) can exacerbate the degree of ototoxicity of a known ototoxin.
- Ototoxicity monitoring is vital when dosing with life-saving ototoxins, especially as any identified hearing loss can then be more rapidly rehabilitated, ameliorating the negative impact of drug-induced hearing loss.

DISCLOSURE

The author has no conflicts of interests pertinent to this article. This review was supported by National Institutes of Health research awards R01 DC004555 and R01 DC016880, as well as an NIGMS CoBRE Award P20 GM139762 to P.S. Steyger.

REFERENCES

1. Gopal KV, Wu C, Shrestha B, et al. D-Methionine protects against cisplatin-induced neurotoxicity in cortical networks. Neurotoxicol Teratol 2012;34(5): 495–504.
2. Hinduja S, Kraus KS, Manohar S, et al. D-methionine protects against cisplatin-induced neurotoxicity in the hippocampus of the adult rat. Neurotox Res 2015; 27(3):199–204.
3. Humes HD. Insights into ototoxicity. Analogies to nephrotoxicity. Ann N Y Acad Sci 1999;884:15–8.

4. Jiang M, Karasawa T, Steyger PS. Aminoglycoside-induced cochleotoxicity: a review. Front Cell Neurosci 2017;11:308.
5. Karasawa T, Steyger PS. An integrated view of cisplatin-induced nephrotoxicity and ototoxicity. Toxicol Lett 2015;237(3):219–27.
6. Wu WJ, Sha SH, McLaren JD, et al. Aminoglycoside ototoxicity in adult CBA, C57BL and BALB mice and the Sprague-Dawley rat. Hear Res 2001; 158(1–2):165–78.
7. Garinis AC, Cross CP, Srikanth P, et al. The cumulative effects of intravenous antibiotic treatments on hearing in patients with cystic fibrosis. J Cyst Fibros 2017;16(3):401–9.
8. Garinis AC, Liao S, Cross CP, et al. Effect of gentamicin and levels of ambient sound on hearing screening outcomes in the neonatal intensive care unit: a pilot study. Int J Pediatr Otorhinolaryngol 2017;97:42–50.
9. Fausti SA, Frey RH, Henry JA, et al. Early detection of ototoxicity using high-frequency, tone-burst-evoked auditory brainstem responses. J Am Acad Audiol 1992;3(6):397–404.
10. Fausti SA, Henry JA, Schaffer HI, et al. High-frequency audiometric monitoring for early detection of aminoglycoside ototoxicity. J Infect Dis 1992;165(6): 1026–32.
11. Elson EC, Meier E, Oermann CM. The implementation of an aminoglycoside induced ototoxicity algorithm for people with cystic fibrosis. J Cyst Fibros 2020;20(2):284–7.
12. Kros CJ, Steyger PS. Aminoglycoside- and cisplatin-induced ototoxicity: mechanisms and otoprotective strategies. Cold Spring Harb Perspect Med 2019; 9(11):a033548.
13. Knight KR, Kraemer DF, Neuwelt EA. Ototoxicity in children receiving platinum chemotherapy: underestimating a commonly occurring toxicity that may influence academic and social development. J Clin Oncol 2005;23(34):8588–96.
14. Knight KR, Kraemer DF, Winter C, et al. Early changes in auditory function as a result of platinum chemotherapy: use of extended high-frequency audiometry and evoked distortion product otoacoustic emissions. J Clin Oncol 2007; 25(10):1190–5.
15. Brock PR, Knight KR, Freyer DR, et al. Platinum-induced ototoxicity in children: a consensus review on mechanisms, predisposition, and protection, including a new International Society of Pediatric Oncology Boston ototoxicity scale. J Clin Oncol 2012;30(19):2408–17.
16. Prayuenyong P, Taylor JA, Pearson SE, et al. Vestibulotoxicity associated with platinum-based chemotherapy in survivors of cancer: a scoping review. Front Oncol 2018;8:363.
17. Callejo A, Durochat A, Bressieux S, et al. Dose-dependent cochlear and vestibular toxicity of trans-tympanic cisplatin in the rat. Neurotoxicology 2017;60:1–9.
18. Crumling MA, King KA, Duncan RK. Cyclodextrins and iatrogenic hearing loss: new drugs with significant risk. Front Cell Neurosci 2017;11:355.
19. Davis RR, Murphy WJ, Snawder JE, et al. Susceptibility to the ototoxic properties of toluene is species specific. Hear Res 2002;166(1–2):24–32.
20. Crofton KM, Lassiter TL, Rebert CS. Solvent-induced ototoxicity in rats: an atypical selective mid- frequency hearing deficit. Hear Res 1994;80(1):25–30.
21. Gagnaire F, Langlais C. Relative ototoxicity of 21 aromatic solvents. Arch Toxicol 2005;79(6):346–54.
22. Counter SA, Buchanan LH. Neuro-ototoxicity in andean adults with chronic lead and noise exposure. J Occup Environ Med 2002;44(1):30–8.

23. Jamesdaniel S, Rosati R, Westrick J, et al. Chronic lead exposure induces cochlear oxidative stress and potentiates noise-induced hearing loss. Toxicol Lett 2018;292:175–80.

24. Hernandez PP, Moreno V, Olivari FA, et al. Sub-lethal concentrations of water-borne copper are toxic to lateral line neuromasts in zebrafish (Danio rerio). Hear Res 2006;213(1–2):1–10.

25. Olivari FA, Hernandez PP, Allende ML. Acute copper exposure induces oxidative stress and cell death in lateral line hair cells of zebrafish larvae. Brain Res 2008;1244:1–12.

26. Dedhia K, Kitsko D, Sabo D, et al. Children with sensorineural hearing loss after passing the newborn hearing screen. JAMA Otolaryngol Head Neck Surg 2013; 139(2):119–23.

27. Gurney JG, Tersak JM, Ness KK, et al. Hearing loss, quality of life, and academic problems in long-term neuroblastoma survivors: a report from the Children's Oncology Group. Pediatrics 2007;120(5):e1229–36.

28. Smith PF, Zheng Y. From ear to uncertainty: vestibular contributions to cognitive function. Front Integr Neurosci 2013;7:84.

29. Smith PF, Darlington CL. Personality changes in patients with vestibular dysfunction. Front Hum Neurosci 2013;7:678.

30. Mohr PE, Feldman JJ, Dunbar JL, et al. The societal costs of severe to profound hearing loss in the United States. Int J Technol Assess Health Care 2000;16(4): 1120–35.

31. Nyberg S, Abbott NJ, Shi X, et al. Delivery of therapeutics to the inner ear: the challenge of the blood-labyrinth barrier. Sci Transl Med 2019;11(482):eaao0935.

32. Tran Ba Huy P, Bernard P, Schacht J. Kinetics of gentamicin uptake and release in the rat. Comparison of inner ear tissues and fluids with other organs. J Clin Invest 1986;77(5):1492–500.

33. Hellberg V, Wallin I, Ehrsson H, et al. Cochlear pharmacokinetics of cisplatin: an in vivo study in the guinea pig. Laryngoscope 2013;123(12):3172–7.

34. Li H, Steyger PS. Systemic aminoglycosides are trafficked via endolymph into cochlear hair cells. Sci Rep 2011;1:159.

35. Breglio AM, Rusheen AE, Shide ED, et al. Cisplatin is retained in the cochlea indefinitely following chemotherapy. Nat Commun 2017;8(1):1654.

36. Chu YH, Sibrian-Vazquez M, Escobedo JO, et al. Systemic delivery and biodistribution of cisplatin in vivo. Mol Pharm 2016;13(8):2677–82.

37. van Ruijven MW, de Groot JC, Hendriksen F, et al. Immunohistochemical detection of platinated DNA in the cochlea of cisplatin-treated guinea pigs. Hear Res 2005;203(1–2):112–21.

38. Koo JW, Quintanilla-Dieck L, Jiang M, et al. Endotoxemia-mediated inflammation potentiates aminoglycoside-induced ototoxicity. Sci Transl Med 2015;7(298): 298ra118.

39. Hiel H, Erre JP, Aurousseau C, et al. Gentamicin uptake by cochlear hair cells precedes hearing impairment during chronic treatment. Audiology 1993;32(1): 78–87.

40. Marcotti W, van Netten SM, Kros CJ. The aminoglycoside antibiotic dihydros-treptomycin rapidly enters mouse outer hair cells through the mechano-electrical transducer channels. J Physiol 2005;567(Pt 2):505–21.

41. Pan B, Akyuz N, Liu XP, et al. TMC1 forms the pore of mechanosensory transduction channels in vertebrate inner ear hair cells. Neuron 2018;99(4): 736–53.e6.

42. Alharazneh A, Luk L, Huth M, et al. Functional hair cell mechanotransducer channels are required for aminoglycoside ototoxicity. PLoS One 2011;6(7): e22347.

43. Coffin AB, Reinhart KE, Owens KN, et al. Extracellular divalent cations modulate aminoglycoside-induced hair cell death in the zebrafish lateral line. Hear Res 2009;253(1–2):42–51.

44. Nilius B, Szallasi A. Transient receptor potential channels as drug targets: from the science of basic research to the art of medicine. Pharmacol Rev 2014;66(3): 676–814.

45. Karasawa T, Wang Q, Fu Y, et al. TRPV4 enhances the cellular uptake of amino-glycoside antibiotics. J Cell Sci 2008;121(Pt 17):2871–9.

46. Myrdal SE, Steyger PS. TRPV1 regulators mediate gentamicin penetration of cultured kidney cells. Hear Res 2005;204(1–2):170–82.

47. Zheng J, Dai C, Steyger PS, et al. Vanilloid receptors in hearing: altered cochlear sensitivity by vanilloids and expression of TRPV1 in the organ of corti. J Neurophysiol 2003;90(1):444–55.

48. Jiang M, Li H, Johnson A, et al. Inflammation up-regulates cochlear expression of TRPV1 to potentiate drug-induced hearing loss. Sci Adv 2019;5(7):eaaw1836.

49. Stepanyan RS, Indzhykulian AA, Velez-Ortega AC, et al. TRPA1-mediated accu-mulation of aminoglycosides in mouse cochlear outer hair cells. J Assoc Res Otolaryngol 2011;12(6):729–40.

50. Vu AA, Nadaraja GS, Huth ME, et al. Integrity and regeneration of mechano-transduction machinery regulate aminoglycoside entry and sensory cell death. PLoS One 2013;8(1):e54794.

51. Hailey DW, Esterberg R, Linbo TH, et al. Fluorescent aminoglycosides reveal intracellular trafficking routes in mechanosensory hair cells. J Clin Invest 2017;127(2):472–86.

52. Hall MD, Okabe M, Shen DW, et al. The role of cellular accumulation in deter-mining sensitivity to platinum-based chemotherapy. Annu Rev Pharmacol Toxi-col 2008;48:495–535.

53. Thomas AJ, Hailey DW, Stawicki TM, et al. Functional mechanotransduction is required for cisplatin-induced hair cell death in the zebrafish lateral line. J Neurosci 2013;33(10):4405–14.

54. Forge A, Schacht J. Aminoglycoside antibiotics. Audiol Neurootol 2000; 5(1):3–22.

55. Prayuenyong P, Baguley D, Kros CJ, et al. Preferential cochleotoxicity of cisplatin. Front Neurosci 2021 (in press).

56. Oh GS, Kim HJ, Choi JH, et al. Activation of lipopolysaccharide-TLR4 signaling accelerates the ototoxic potential of cisplatin in mice. J Immunol 2011;186(2): 1140–50.

57. Qian X, He Z, Wang Y, et al. Hair cell uptake of gentamicin in the developing mouse utricle. J Cell Physiol 2021;236(7):5235–52.

58. Cross CP, Liao S, Urdang ZD, et al. Effect of sepsis and systemic inflammatory response syndrome on neonatal hearing screening outcomes following genta-micin exposure. Int J Pediatr Otorhinolaryngol 2015;79(11):1915–9.

59. Henry KR, Guess MB, Chole RA. Hyperthermia increases aminoglycoside ototoxicity. Acta Otolaryngol 1983;95(3–4):323–7.

60. Kaplanski G, Granel B, Vaz T, et al. Jarisch-Herxheimer reaction complicating the treatment of chronic Q fever endocarditis: elevated TNFalpha and IL-6 serum levels. The J Infect 1998;37(1):83–4.

61. Shenep JL, Mogan KA. Kinetics of endotoxin release during antibiotic therapy for experimental gram-negative bacterial sepsis. J Infect Dis 1984;150(3): 380–8.

62. Coffin AB, Boney R, Hill JD, et al. Detecting novel ototoxins and potentiation of ototoxicity by disease settings. Front Neurol 2021 (in press).

63. Jiang M, Taghizadeh F, Steyger PS. Potential mechanisms underlying inflammation-enhanced aminoglycoside-induced cochleotoxicity. Front Cell Neurosci 2017;11:362.

64. Zager RA. Endotoxemia, renal hypoperfusion, and fever: interactive risk factors for aminoglycoside and sepsis-associated acute renal failure. Am J Kidney Dis 1992;20(3):223–30.

65. Gandara DR, Perez EA, Weibe V, et al. Cisplatin chemoprotection and rescue: pharmacologic modulation of toxicity. Semin Oncol 1991;18(1 Suppl 3):49–55.

66. Gatell JM, Ferran F, Araujo V, et al. Univariate and multivariate analyses of risk factors predisposing to auditory toxicity in patients receiving aminoglycosides. Antimicrob Agents Chemother 1987;31(9):1383–7.

67. Manian FA, Stone WJ, Alford RH. Adverse antibiotic effects associated with renal insufficiency. Rev Infect Dis 1990;12(2):236–49.

68. McClure CL. Common infections in the elderly. Am Fam Physician 1992;45(6): 2691–8.

69. Triggs E, Charles B. Pharmacokinetics and therapeutic drug monitoring of gentamicin in the elderly. Clin Pharmacokinet 1999;37(4):331–41.

70. Lautermann J, McLaren J, Schacht J. Glutathione protection against gentamicin ototoxicity depends on nutritional status. Hear Res 1995;86(1–2):15–24.

71. Lautermann J, Crann SA, McLaren J, et al. Glutathione-dependent antioxidant systems in the mammalian inner ear: effects of aging, ototoxic drugs and noise. Hear Res 1997;114(1–2):75–82.

72. Lautermann J, Song B, McLaren J, et al. Diet is a risk factor in cisplatin ototoxicity. Hear Res 1995;88(1–2):47–53.

73. Spankovich C, Lobarinas E, Ding D, et al. Assessment of thermal treatment via irrigation of external ear to reduce cisplatin-induced hearing loss. Hear Res 2016;332:55–60.

74. Lin CD, Kao MC, Tsai MH, et al. Transient ischemia/hypoxia enhances gentamicin ototoxicity via caspase-dependent cell death pathway. Lab Invest 2011; 91(7):1092–106.

75. McKinney W, Yonovitz A, Smolensky MH. Circadian variation of gentamicin toxicity in rats. Laryngoscope 2015;125(7):E252–6.

76. Soulban G, Smolensky MH, Yonovitz A. Gentamicin-induced chronotoxicity: use of body temperature as a circadian marker rhythm. Chronobiol Int 1990;7(5–6): 393–402.

77. Bielefeld EC, Markle A, DeBacker JR, et al. Chronotolerance for cisplatin ototoxicity in the rat. Hear Res 2018;370:16–21.

78. Tserga E, Moreno-Paublete R, Sarlus H, et al. Circadian vulnerability of cisplatin-induced ototoxicity in the cochlea. FASEB J 2020;34(10):13978–92.

79. Hobbie SN, Bruell CM, Akshay S, et al. Mitochondrial deafness alleles confer misreading of the genetic code. Proc Natl Acad Sci U S A 2008;105(9):3244–9.

80. Qian Y, Guan MX. Interaction of aminoglycosides with human mitochondrial 12S rRNA carrying the deafness-associated mutation. Antimicrob Agents Chemother 2009;53(11):4612–8.

81. Matt T, Ng CL, Lang K, et al. Dissociation of antibacterial activity and aminogly-coside ototoxicity in the 4-monosubstituted 2-deoxystreptamine apramycin. Proc Natl Acad Sci U S A 2012;109(27):10984–9.

82. McDermott JH, Wolf J, Hoshitsuki K, et al. Clinical Pharmacogenetics Implementation Consortium (CPIC) guideline for the use of aminoglycosides based on MT-RNR1 genotype. J Neuroinflammation 2021;18(1):16.

83. Turan C, Kantar M, Aktan C, et al. Cisplatin ototoxicity in children: risk factors and its relationship with polymorphisms of DNA repair genes ERCC1, ERCC2, and XRCC1. Cancer Chemother Pharmacol 2019;84(6):1333–8.

84. Caronia D, Patino-Garcia A, Milne RL, et al. Common variations in ERCC2 are associated with response to cisplatin chemotherapy and clinical outcome in osteosarcoma patients. Pharmacogenomics J 2009;9(5):347–53.

85. Xu H, Robinson GW, Huang J, et al. Common variants in ACYP2 influence susceptibility to cisplatin-induced hearing loss. Nat Genet 2015;47(3):263–6.

86. Ross CJ, Katzov-Eckert H, Dube MP, et al. Genetic variants in TPMT and COMT are associated with hearing loss in children receiving cisplatin chemotherapy. Nat Genet 2009;41(12):1345–9.

87. Langer T, Clemens E, Broer L, et al. Usefulness of current candidate genetic markers to identify childhood cancer patients at risk for platinum-induced ototoxicity: results of the European PanCareLIFE cohort study. Eur J Cancer 2020;138:212–24.

88. Tserga E, Nandwani T, Edvall NK, et al. The genetic vulnerability to cisplatin ototoxicity: a systematic review. Sci Rep 2019;9(1):3455.

89. Masumoto K, Nagata K, Uesugi T, et al. Risk factors for sensorineural hearing loss in survivors with severe congenital diaphragmatic hernia. Eur J Pediatr 2007;166(6):607–12.

90. Cheung PY, Tyebkhan JM, Peliowski A, et al. Prolonged use of pancuronium bromide and sensorineural hearing loss in childhood survivors of congenital diaphragmatic hernia. J Pediatr 1999;135(2 Pt 1):233–9.

91. Mathog RH, Klein WJ Jr. Ototoxicity of ethacrynic acid and aminoglycoside antibiotics in uremia. N Engl J Med 1969;280(22):1223–4.

92. Rybak LP. Ototoxicity of loop diuretics. Otolaryngol Clin North Am 1993;26(5):829–44.

93. Bates DE, Beaumont SJ, Baylis BW. Ototoxicity induced by gentamicin and furosemide. Ann Pharmacother 2002;36(3):446–51.

94. Rubin LG, Sanchez PJ, Siegel J, et al. Evaluation and treatment of neonates with suspected late-onset sepsis: a survey of neonatologists' practices. Pediatrics 2002;110(4):e42.

95. Brummett RE, Fox KE, Jacobs F, et al. Augmented gentamicin ototoxicity induced by vancomycin in guinea pigs. Arch Otolaryngol Head Neck Surg 1990;116(1):61–4.

96. Clemens E, de Vries AC, Pluijm SF, et al. Determinants of ototoxicity in 451 platinum-treated Dutch survivors of childhood cancer: a DCOG late-effects study. Eur J Cancer 2016;69:77–85.

97. McAlpine D, Johnstone BM. The ototoxic mechanism of cisplatin. Hear Res 1990;47(3):191–203.

98. Miller MW, Riedel G, Hoistad D, et al. Ototoxicity after combined platinum and fractionated radiation in a novel guinea pig model. Am J Otolaryngol 2009;30(1):1–7.

99. Paulino AC, Lobo M, Teh BS, et al. Ototoxicity after intensity-modulated radiation therapy and cisplatin-based chemotherapy in children with medulloblastoma. Int J Radiat Oncol Biol Phys 2010;78(5):1445–50.

100. Collins PW. Synergistic interactions of gentamicin and pure tones causing cochlear hair cell loss in pigmented guinea pigs. Hear Res 1988;36(2–3): 249–59.

101. Li H, Steyger PS. Synergistic ototoxicity due to noise exposure and aminoglycoside antibiotics. Noise Health 2009;11(42):26–32.

102. Steyger PS. Mechanisms of aminoglycoside- and cisplatin-induced ototoxicity. Am J Audiol 2021;1–14 [Epub ahead of print].

103. Gratton MA, Salvi RJ, Kamen BA, et al. Interaction of cisplatin and noise on the peripheral auditory system. Hear Res 1990;50(1–2):211–23.

104. Bokemeyer C, Berger CC, Hartmann JT, et al. Analysis of risk factors for cisplatin-induced ototoxicity in patients with testicular cancer. Br J Cancer 1998;77(8):1355–62.

105. Laurell GF. Combined effects of noise and cisplatin: short- and long-term follow-up. Ann Otol Rhinol Laryngol 1992;101(12):969–76.

106. DeBacker JR, Harrison RT, Bielefeld EC. Long-term synergistic interaction of cisplatin- and noise-induced hearing losses. Ear Hear 2017;38(3):282–91.

107. Huth ME, Ricci AJ, Cheng AG. Mechanisms of aminoglycoside ototoxicity and targets of hair cell protection. Int J Otolaryngol 2011;2011:937861.

108. Sheth S, Mukherjea D, Rybak LP, et al. Mechanisms of cisplatin-induced ototoxicity and otoprotection. Front Cell Neurosci 2017;11:338.

109. Huth ME, Han KH, Sotoudeh K, et al. Designer aminoglycosides prevent cochlear hair cell loss and hearing loss. J Clin Invest 2015;125(2):583–92.

110. O'Sullivan ME, Song Y, Greenhouse R, et al. Dissociating antibacterial from ototoxic effects of gentamicin C-subtypes. Proc Natl Acad Sci U S A 2020; 117(51):32423–32.

111. Salt AN, Plontke SK. Principles of local drug delivery to the inner ear. Audiol Neurootol 2009;14(6):350–60.

112. Ramaswamy B, Roy S, Apolo AB, et al. Magnetic nanoparticle mediated steroid delivery mitigates cisplatin induced hearing loss. Front Cell Neurosci 2017; 11:268.

113. Hammann F, Schoning V, Drewe J. Prediction of clinically relevant drug-induced liver injury from structure using machine learning. J Appl Toxicol 2019;39(3): 412–9.

114. Cai C, Guo P, Zhou Y, et al. Deep learning-based prediction of drug-induced cardiotoxicity. J Chem Inf Model 2019;59(3):1073–84.

115. Ryals M, Morell RJ, Martin D, et al. The inner ear heat shock transcriptional signature identifies compounds that protect against aminoglycoside ototoxicity. Front Cell Neurosci 2018;12:445.

116. Kalinec GM, Webster P, Lim DJ, et al. A cochlear cell line as an in vitro system for drug ototoxicity screening. Audiol Neurootol 2003;8(4):177–89.

117. Ingersoll MA, Malloy EA, Caster LE, et al. BRAF inhibition protects against hearing loss in mice. Sci Adv 2020;6(49):eabd0561.

118. Teitz T, Fang J, Goktug AN, et al. CDK2 inhibitors as candidate therapeutics for cisplatin- and noise-induced hearing loss. J Exp Med 2018;215(4):1187–203.

119. Hazlitt RA, Teitz T, Bonga JD, et al. Development of second-generation CDK2 inhibitors for the prevention of cisplatin-induced hearing loss. J Med Chem 2018;61(17):7700–9.

120. Karasawa T, Wang Q, David LL, et al. CLIMP-63 is a gentamicin-binding protein that is involved in drug-induced cytotoxicity. Cell Death Dis 2010;1:e102.
121. Karasawa T, Wang Q, David LL, et al. Calreticulin binds to gentamicin and reduces drug-induced ototoxicity. Toxicol Sci 2011;124(2):378–87.
122. Harris JA, Cheng AG, Cunningham LL, et al. Neomycin-induced hair cell death and rapid regeneration in the lateral line of zebrafish (Danio rerio). J Assoc Res Otolaryngol 2003;4(2):219–34.
123. Owens KN, Santos F, Roberts B, et al. Identification of genetic and chemical modulators of zebrafish mechanosensory hair cell death. PLoS Genet 2008; 4(2):e1000020.
124. Chowdhury S, Owens KN, Herr RJ, et al. Phenotypic optimization of urea-thiophene carboxamides to yield potent, well tolerated, and orally active protective agents against aminoglycoside-induced hearing loss. J Med Chem 2018; 61(1):84–97.
125. Kenyon EJ, Kirkwood NK, Kitcher SR, et al. Identification of ion-channel modulators that protect against aminoglycoside-induced hair cell death. JCI Insight 2017;2(24):e96773.
126. Karasawa T, Sibrian-Vazquez M, Strongin RM, et al. Identification of cisplatin-binding proteins using agarose conjugates of platinum compounds. PLoS One 2013;8(6):e66220.
127. Dai CF, Mangiardi D, Cotanche DA, et al. Uptake of fluorescent gentamicin by vertebrate sensory cells in vivo. Hear Res 2006;213(1–2):64–78.
128. Fernandez K, Spielbauer KK, Rusheen A, et al. Lovastatin protects against cisplatin-induced hearing loss in mice. Hear Res 2020;389:107905.
129. Fernandez KA, Allen P, Campbell M, et al. Atorvastatin is associated with reduced cisplatin-induced hearing loss. J Clin Invest 2021;131(1):e142616.
130. Trung NT, Hien TT, Huyen TT, et al. Enrichment of bacterial DNA for the diagnosis of blood stream infections. BMC Infect Dis 2016;16:235.
131. Jing W, Zongjie H, Denggang F, et al. Mitochondrial mutations associated with aminoglycoside ototoxicity and hearing loss susceptibility identified by meta-analysis. J Med Genet 2015;52(2):95–103.
132. Garinis AC, Poling GL, Rubenstein RC, et al. Clinical considerations for routine auditory and vestibular monitoring in patients with cystic fibrosis. Am J Audiol 2021. in press.

Early Identification and Management of Congenital Cytomegalovirus

Carolyn M. Jenks, MD[a], Leena B. Mithal, MD, MSCI[b,c],
Stephen R. Hoff, MD[d,e],*

KEYWORDS

- Congenital cytomegalovirus • Congenital CMV • Hearing loss • Valganciclovir

KEY POINTS

- Congenital cytomegalovirus (cCMV) is the most common nongenetic cause of sensorineural hearing loss.
- There is no universal screening for cCMV. Therefore, it is often not diagnosed in children who are otherwise asymptomatic.
- Hearing loss owing to cCMV is often delayed in onset, is progressive, and can be bilateral or unilateral.
- Children with cCMV with severe to profound sensorineural hearing loss in one or both ears are potential candidates for cochlear implant.

INTRODUCTION

Congenital cytomegalovirus (cCMV) is the most common intrauterine infection, resulting in an overall birth prevalence of approximately 0.7%.[1,2] Prevalence varies among populations and is considerably higher in the developing world.[3] The most common manifestation of cCMV is sensorineural hearing loss (SNHL), and for this reason, cCMV is the most common nongenetic cause of SNHL, accounting for approximately one-quarter of early childhood SNHL.[4,5] The recognition of cCMV as a cause of SNHL is underestimated in clinical practice because (1) most of the affected children are otherwise asymptomatic and therefore not tested and diagnosed with cCMV at birth;

[a] Department Otolaryngology–Head & Neck Surgery, Johns Hopkins University School of Medicine, 601 North Caroline Street 6th Floor, Baltimore, MD 21287, USA; [b] Department of Pediatrics, Division of Infectious Diseases, Northwestern University Feinberg School of Medicine, Chicago, IL, USA; [c] Ann & Robert H. Lurie Children's Hospital of Chicago, 225 East Chicago Avenue, Box #20, Chicago, IL 60611, USA; [d] Department Otolaryngology–Head & Neck Surgery, Northwestern University Feinberg School of Medicine, Chicago, IL, USA; [e] Division of Otolaryngology–Head & Neck Surgery, Ann & Robert H. Lurie Children's Hospital of Chicago, 225 East Chicago Avenue, Chicago, IL 60611, USA
* Corresponding author.
E-mail address: shoff@luriechildrens.org

Otolaryngol Clin N Am 54 (2021) 1117–1127
https://doi.org/10.1016/j.otc.2021.06.006
0030-6665/21/© 2021 Elsevier Inc. All rights reserved.

and (2) delayed onset of hearing loss is common with onset after the period within which definitive diagnosis can be made. This article aims to provide an overview of cCMV transmission, manifestations, and management of cCMV and its associated SNHL.

TRANSMISSION OF CYTOMEGALOVIRUS

Cytomegalovirus (CMV) is a member of the herpesvirus family and is highly prevalent, infecting many people by childhood or early adulthood worldwide.[6] Prevalence among women of reproductive age is estimated at 79% in North America and 86% globally.[7] Infection spreads through contact with infected bodily fluids, including urine, saliva, blood, or genital secretions. Repeated reinfection with CMV is common. Infections generally cause mild symptoms, except in those with compromised immune systems and in the case of the developing fetus. Intrauterine transmission occurs because of primary (new) maternal infection or nonprimary infection in seropositive mothers who previously experienced CMV infection. Primary infection, although less common, confers a 40% risk of transmission to the fetus, whereas nonprimary infection confers a 1% to 2% risk. There is no universally recommended CMV screening of mothers during pregnancy and, to date, no proven intervention to decrease transmission to a fetus.

MANIFESTATIONS OF CONGENITAL CYTOMEGALOVIRUS

Manifestations of cCMV are highly variable and range from no apparent sequelae to multisystem involvement. Approximately 10% of cases are symptomatic at birth. The remaining 90% of infections are considered asymptomatic.[1,2] The central nervous system is commonly affected in symptomatic cases and can result in microcephaly, cortical malformations, developmental delay, cerebral palsy, and visual impairment. Additional systemic manifestations include hepatosplenomegaly, hyperbilirubinemia, petechiae, thrombocytopenia, and anemia, findings of which should prompt evaluation for cCMV. cCMV infection is associated with prematurity, low birth weight, and intrauterine growth restriction (IUGR). SNHL is the most common sequela of cCMV. If SNHL is the only symptom in a child with cCMV, these patients have traditionally been referred to in the literature as members of an "asymptomatic" subgroup.

HEARING LOSS

SNHL occurs in 20% to 65% of symptomatic cases and 6% to 25% of asymptomatic cases.[8,9] Among symptomatic cases of cCMV, IUGR, petechiae, microcephaly, and abnormal neuroimaging findings have been associated with SNHL.[10-13] Among asymptomatic cases, prematurity and low birth weight are associated with SNHL.[8,14,15] Increased risk of SNHL has also been found in infants with higher viral load at diagnosis.[16,17] Despite these findings, there is no reliable way to predict which children with symptomatic and asymptomatic cCMV will develop SNHL.

Hearing loss varies from mild to profound and can be unilateral or bilateral, with most children ultimately progressing to severe or profound SNHL.[18-20] The most common audiometric configurations are flat and down-sloping SNHL.[19,20] Hearing loss in symptomatic children tends to be more severe and more often bilateral than in asymptomatic children.[18,21,22]

Hearing loss can be stable, progressive, fluctuating, or rarely, might improve over time. Progression of hearing loss occurs in many (over 50%) of both symptomatic and asymptomatic patients.[18,23,24] Progression can occur at any time, even after years of stability, necessitating long-term audiological follow-up in all patients with cCMV-related hearing loss. In 1 study, progression was first documented on average 51 months (range, 3–186) after diagnosis for asymptomatic infections and 26 months (range, 2–209) for symptomatic infections. Fluctuating hearing loss is also common.[18,23]

Onset of hearing loss is delayed in up to 50% of patients.[25] Median age of onset of delayed hearing loss in a large observational study was 33 months (range, 6–197) and 44 months (range, 24–182) for asymptomatic and symptomatic cases, respectively.[18] In addition, cCMV patients with unilateral hearing loss are at risk of developing SNHL in the contralateral ear.[9]

DIAGNOSTIC TESTING FOR CONGENITAL CYTOMEGALOVIRUS

Testing for cCMV should be done within the first 3 weeks of life to conclusively distinguish congenital infection from postnatally acquired infection. As there is no universal screening for cCMV, prompt testing of children who do not pass newborn screening in one or both ears would identify cCMV in children with SNHL at birth. Viral CMV cultures have been replaced by CMV DNA polymerase chain reaction (PCR) of saliva or urine. Saliva is the simplest to obtain but has more false positive results than urine testing. A positive saliva PCR should be confirmed with a repeat PCR test (preferably urine), ideally within the neonatal period. For children who have not undergone neonatal PCR testing within the optimal time window for accurate testing, another approach is to perform CMV PCR testing on the dried blood spot (DBS). The DBS is routinely collected at birth on all children to screen for a series of disorders and stored by state health departments for varying time periods. Previous studies have reported lower sensitivity of cCMV diagnosis based on blood spot testing, but more recent studies show improved sensitivity.[26,27] Thus, PCR testing of stored DBS might be a useful retrospective means of determining if SNHL and other symptoms are related to cCMV.

TARGETED AND HEARING TARGETED SCREENING

A "targeted screening" approach to cCMV testing is currently in use in some locations wherein infants with symptoms that could be related to cCMV undergo PCR testing. Indications for cCMV testing include thrombocytopenia, transaminitis, conjugated hyperbilirubinemia, IUGR, small for gestational age, microcephaly, rash consistent with cCMV, abnormal head ultrasound with ventriculomegaly or periventricular calcification, hepatosplenomegaly, known maternal infection during pregnancy, and SNHL. Although SNHL as an isolated symptom is not defined as symptomatic cCMV, isolated SNHL is included as an indication for targeted screening given the frequency of which cCMV causes SNHL and the implications for management. The approach to routine cCMV screening in infants with a failed newborn hearing screen (unilateral or bilateral) is referred to as hearing-targeted early cytomegalovirus (HT-CMV) screening. In 2013, Utah became the first state to legislate that CMV testing be accomplished by age 3 weeks for infants who fail newborn hearing screening. Since then, a growing number of medical centers have voluntarily adopted similar institutional policy, and more states have instituted legislation requiring discussion of cCMV testing with parents. HT-CMV policies are useful but do not identify the significant number of children with delayed onset of SNHL owing to cCMV.

BENEFIT OF UNIVERSAL CONGENITAL CYTOMEGALOVIRUS NEWBORN SCREENING

Implementation of targeted screening for cCMV in combination with universal newborn hearing screening has resulted in improved early detection of cCMV-related SNHL. However, as noted previously, a significant proportion of cases will be missed because of delayed presentation of hearing loss beyond the newborn period.[25] For this reason, many experts advocate for universal newborn cCMV screening.[28–30] Universal cCMV screening of all newborns, independent of hearing screening or evidence of symptomatic disease, would enable audiologic monitoring of children at risk of developing SNHL because of this congenital infection. Because early diagnosis and treatment of hearing loss positively impact language, universal cCMV screening has the potential to benefit those children at risk for SNHL.

COMPREHENSIVE EVALUATION OF INFANTS DIAGNOSED WITH CONGENITAL CYTOMEGALOVIRUS

Infants with cCMV, with or without SNHL, benefit from a comprehensive evaluation (**Box 1**) that includes brain imaging by ultrasound or MRI. Characteristic findings include intracranial calcifications, ventriculomegaly, cerebral and cerebellar volume loss, and white matter disease. Findings might be useful in confirming diagnosis of cCMV, in guiding counseling about prognosis, and in identifying candidates for antiviral treatment. In addition, newly diagnosed infants should have laboratory testing to assess for cytopenia and hepatitis and ophthalmologic evaluation to rule out ocular manifestations of cCMV.

COOCCURRENCE OF CONGENITAL CYTOMEGALOVIRUS AND GENETIC CAUSE OF HEARING LOSS

In light of the relatively high incidence of cCMV in the general population, there is reason for concern that it could cooccur with genetic causes of SNHL, which are

---

Box 1
Evaluation, treatment, and monitoring of infants with congenital cytomegalovirus infection

Initial evaluation:
- Diagnosis by saliva or urine CMV PCR within the first 3 weeks of life (positive saliva followed by confirmatory urine) or positive DBS CMV PCR
- If cCMV diagnosed:
    Brain imaging (US or MRI), ophthalmology examination, hearing assessment, laboratory tests (cytopenias hepatitis, kidney function), consider consultation with Infectious Diseases

Antiviral therapy candidates:
- Infants with moderate to severe symptomatic cCMV
- Consider mildly symptomatic infants/isolated SNHL on case-by-case basis

Initiation of treatment:
- Ideally within first month of life

Treatment regimen:
- Oral valganciclovir 16 mg/kg/dose twice daily

Duration of treatment:
- 6 months

Monitoring during treatment:
- Absolute neutrophil counts followed closely (weekly to biweekly) for first 2 months, then monthly for the duration of therapy
- Transaminases and kidney function monthly for the duration of therapy

Follow-up as indicated:
- Ophthalmology
- Audiology (see **Fig. 1**) and Otolaryngology
- Case-by-case: Infectious Diseases, Neurology, developmental assessment, and therapy

Abbreviation: US, ultrasound.

known to account for more than half of childhood hearing loss. This raises the question of whether children with cCMV diagnosed with bilateral SNHL should also undergo comprehensive genetic testing. To date, cooccurrence of genetic causes of hearing loss has been reported in a small percentage of this population.[31,32] However, consensus on the genetic testing for children with bilateral SNHL and cCMV is currently lacking.

HEARING LOSS SCREENING AND MONITORING

Although only a minority of children with cCMV develop SNHL, prediction of which children will develop hearing loss is not possible. Therefore, it is necessary that children known to have cCMV infection receive ongoing audiologic surveillance (**Fig. 1**). The Joint Committee on Infant Hearing has stated that "early and more frequent assessment" might be indicated for children with cCMV infection as compared with their recommendation of "at least one" additional audiology assessment by 24 to 30 months of age for children who pass newborn hearing screening but have risk factors for hearing loss.[33] Other monitoring recommendations for delayed onset of hearing loss in children with cCMV vary from every 6 to 12 months until age 4 to 6 years (see **Fig. 1**).[4,20,34] The risk of delayed-onset SNHL is reported to return to a level comparable to non-cCMV-infected controls by age 5 years.[9] Children with cCMV and confirmed SNHL, whether onset is at birth or delayed, require ongoing audiologic

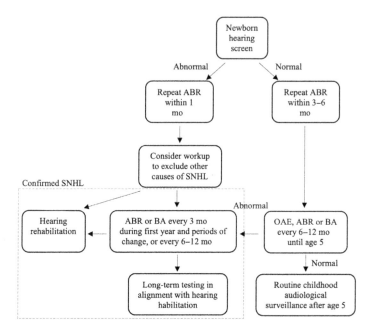

Fig. 1. Flowchart of hearing screening and monitoring in patients with cCMV. ABR, auditory brainstem response; BA, behavioral audiometry; OAE, otoacoustic emissions. (*Adapted from* Foulon I, Vleurinck L, Kerkhofs K, Gordts F. Hearing configuration in children with ccmv infection and proposal of a flow chart for hearing evaluation.Int J Audiol. 2015;54(10):714-9. copyright ©BritishSociety of Audiology; International Society of Audiology; Nordic Audiological Society, reprinted by permissionof Informa UK Limited, trading as Taylor & Francis Group, www.tandfonline.com on behalf of British Society of Audiology; International Society of Audiology; Nordic Audiological Society.)

monitoring for stability of hearing loss and management. To optimize amplification, more frequent audiologic testing is often necessary during the first year of life and during periods whereby hearing is fluctuating or progressing.[4,20]

Techniques used to screen for hearing loss and to perform diagnostic audiologic evaluations will vary based on the age and development of the patient (see **Fig. 1**). Evaluation and management by an experienced pediatric audiologist are ideal. Auditory brainstem response testing is necessary for young infants, as well as older children who are difficult to test by behavioral techniques. Further information on audiologic approach to diagnosis of hearing loss in children can be found in Linda J. Hood's article, "Auditory Neuropathy / Auditory Synaptopathy," in this issue.

MANAGEMENT OF SENSORINEURAL HEARING LOSS

Hearing habilitation should be pursued for children with SNHL, regardless of cause, to minimize the impact of hearing loss on speech, language, and cognition. The first line of treatment is amplification for children with bilateral SNHL or unilateral SNHL of mild to moderate degree (see Sampat Sindhar and Judith E.C. Lieu's article, "Overview of Medical Evaluation of Unilateral & Bilateral Hearing Loss in Children," in this issue). Amplification should not be delayed by antiviral treatment. To maximize listening and spoken language, early intervention therapy that includes listening and spoken language therapy is beneficial.

COCHLEAR IMPLANTATION

Cochlear implantation (CI) is the only medical treatment of SNHL when amplification does not provide adequate access to spoken language. Benefits of CI in patients with cCMV are well established, with multiple series showing improvement in auditory thresholds, speech perception, and expression.[32,35–40] Some studies have shown equivalent progress among implanted patients with cCMV compared with controls with other causes of SNHL, whereas others have shown comparatively slower or poorer progress.[32,36,38,39,41]

Children with cCMV, especially those with symptomatic cCMV, can have comorbidities and developmental delays placing them at increased risk for cognitive impairment. In the past, children with these comorbidities have been viewed as poor candidates for CI. However, CI candidacy has evolved to include children with significant additional disabilities, and the benefits have been well established.[42–44] Early access to CI can be critical to these children to fully develop their hearing, language, and cognitive potential.

For children with cCMV and single-sided deafness, or asymmetric hearing loss with severe to profound loss in 1 ear, CI is also a consideration. Having useful hearing from only 1 ear is associated with many disadvantages, including increased difficulty hearing in background noise and poor sound localization. The risk of progression or onset of hearing loss in the better hearing ear also makes early implantation of the poorer ear more compelling. In addition, for the subpopulation of children with symptomatic cCMV who also have visual impairment, improvement of hearing is especially important.[13,45]

ANTIVIRAL TREATMENT FOR CONGENITAL CYTOMEGALOVIRUS

Over the last 3 decades, antiviral medications have emerged as a viable treatment option. Several early studies of children with symptomatic CMV treated with 6 weeks of intravenous ganciclovir provided promising evidence of positive impact on hearing preservation in the short term.[46,47] In addition, antiviral treatment might also improve neurodevelopmental outcomes.[48] The most significant risk of antiviral treatment is significant neutropenia, which is dose-dependent and reversible. Possible side effects of antiviral therapy include thrombocytopenia, anemia, and kidney and liver dysfunction.

Valganciclovir is an orally administered antiviral medication that has supplanted ganciclovir as the drug of choice for treatment of symptomatic cCMV. It offers equivalent pharmacokinetics, ease of oral administration, and a lower side-effect profile.[49,50] A 6-month course of oral treatment is more effective to optimize hearing outcomes than 6 weeks of therapy. Neutropenia occurs less frequently with oral than with intravenous antiviral treatment.[51] In some cases, improvement in auditory thresholds has been noted, more commonly in ears with less hearing loss. In addition, infants treated with 6 months of oral valganciclovir have been found to have improved neurodevelopmental scores at 24 months.[51]

It is standard care to offer antiviral treatment (see **Box 1**) for infants with moderate to severe symptomatic cCMV.[52] Moderately to severely symptomatic cCMV disease includes infants with multiple manifestations of cCMV disease or who have central nervous system involvement beyond SNHL. Treatment should ideally be initiated within the first month of life, and standard length of treatment is 6 months. Whether there is also benefit when treatment is initiated after the first month of life is an area of active study.[53,54]

Several trials are underway to determine the benefit of antiviral therapy for asymptomatic cCMV, with and without SNHL, and the timing of treatment initiation (ClinicalTrials.gov Identifiers: NCT01649869, NCT03107871, NCT03301415). Results of these studies might support expanded indications and windows for treatment.

At the Ann and Robert H. Lurie Children's Hospital of Chicago, antiviral therapy is offered on a case-by-case basis to children with mild symptomatic or asymptomatic disease with SNHL. Children are comprehensively evaluated by their Infectious Disease specialists (see **Box 1**) and counseled as to the potential benefits and risks of oral antiviral therapy and required monitoring. Ideally, these children are treated within the setting of a clinical trial; however, treatment is offered outside of a trial for those who do not qualify or decline participation. The primary goal of antiviral therapy in these children is stabilization of hearing loss as well as prevention of hearing loss in the normal hearing ear, if present. In discussing antiviral therapy, parents are informed about (1) current level of evidence of treatment effectiveness, (2) applicability to the individual child's history, and (3) potential known and unknown side effects.

SUMMARY

cCMV is the most common nongenetic cause of SNHL. Hearing loss caused by cCMV is often bilateral but can be asymmetric or unilateral and of varying degree. Children with cCMV may pass newborn hearing screening because almost half present with delayed onset of hearing loss. Those with residual hearing are at significant risk for progression and, therefore, require careful audiologic monitoring. The role of antiviral therapy to address SNHL in children with otherwise mild or asymptomatic disease is emerging. Children with cCMV and significant SNHL in one or both ears may be excellent candidates for CI.

CLINICS CARE POINTS

- Targeted hearing screening for congenital cytomegalovirus with polymerase chain reaction testing completed before 3 weeks of age for infants who fail newborn hearing screening is an effective policy to increase diagnosis of congenital cytomegalovirus–related sensorineural hearing loss. This approach also enables the option of antiviral therapy to preserve hearing for this population.

- Children with congenital cytomegalovirus–related sensorineural hearing loss require monitoring for progression of hearing loss and appropriate hearing technology to address their unilateral or bilateral loss in order to maximize language and developmental outcome.

- Congenital cytomegalovirus should be considered as a possible cause of postnatal sensorineural hearing loss. Definitive diagnosis of congenital cytomegalovirus as the cause of postnatal sensorineural hearing loss might not be possible beyond the neonatal period and especially in otherwise asymptomatic children unless polymerase chain reaction testing of the dried blood spot is positive. However, at this time, children with delayed onset sensorineural hearing loss are not candidates for antiviral therapy because evidence of benefit to hearing or overall development is lacking for treatment initiated after the neonatal period.

- Cochlear implantation is an effective treatment for congenital cytomegalovirus–related sensorineural hearing loss when amplification does not provide access to spoken language. Candidates include children with complicating conditions and developmental delays in addition to hearing loss. The benefit of binaural hearing provided by an implant for children with congenital cytomegalovirus–related single-sided deafness is also of consideration, especially given the risk for sensorineural hearing loss in the only hearing ear.

DISCLOSURE

Dr L.B. Mithal and Dr S.R. Hoff are site investigators in the ValEAR Trial, NIH U01 DC014706 (PI: Park).

REFERENCES

1. Kenneson A, Cannon MJ. Review and meta-analysis of the epidemiology of congenital cytomegalovirus (CMV) infection. Rev Med Virol 2007;17(4):253–76.
2. Dollard SC, Grosse SD, Ross DS. New estimates of the prevalence of neurological and sensory sequelae and mortality associated with congenital cytomegalovirus infection. Rev Med Virol 2007;17(5):355–63.
3. Lanzieri TM, Dollard SC, Bialek SR, et al. Systematic review of the birth prevalence of congenital cytomegalovirus infection in developing countries. Int J Infect Dis 2014;22:44–8.
4. Fowler KB. Congenital cytomegalovirus infection: audiologic outcome. Clin Infect Dis 2013;57(Suppl 4):S182–4.
5. Morton CC, Nance WE. Newborn hearing screening–a silent revolution. N Engl J Med 2006;354(20):2151–64.
6. Manicklal S, Emery VC, Lazzarotto T, et al. The "silent" global burden of congenital cytomegalovirus. Clin Microbiol Rev 2013;26(1):86–102.
7. Zuhair M, Smit GSA, Wallis G, et al. Estimation of the worldwide seroprevalence of cytomegalovirus: a systematic review and meta-analysis. Rev Med Virol 2019; 29(3):e2034.
8. Fowler KB, Boppana SB. Congenital cytomegalovirus (CMV) infection and hearing deficit. J Clin Virol 2006;35(2):226–31.
9. Lanzieri TM, Chung W, Flores M, et al. Hearing loss in children with asymptomatic congenital cytomegalovirus infection. Pediatrics 2017;139(3):e20162610.
10. Ito Y, Kimura H, Torii Y, et al. Risk factors for poor outcome in congenital cytomegalovirus infection and neonatal herpes on the basis of a nationwide survey in Japan. Pediatr Int 2013;55(5):566–71.

11. Boppana SB, Fowler KB, Vaid Y, et al. Neuroradiographic findings in the newborn period and long-term outcome in children with symptomatic congenital cytomegalovirus infection. Pediatrics 1997;99(3):409–14.

12. Rivera LB, Boppana SB, Fowler KB, et al. Predictors of hearing loss in children with symptomatic congenital cytomegalovirus infection. Pediatrics 2002;110(4): 762–7.

13. Lanzieri TM, Leung J, Caviness AC, et al. Long-term outcomes of children with symptomatic congenital cytomegalovirus disease. J Perinatol 2017;37(7):875–80.

14. Fowler K. Do perinatal factors predict hearing loss in children with asymptomatic congenital (CMV) infection? Am J Epidemiol 2003;157:S84.

15. Dimopoulou D, Kourlaba G, Antoniadou A, et al. Low birth weight and head circumference as potential biomarkers of sensorineural hearing loss in asymptomatic congenitally CMV-infected infants. J Clin Virol 2020;129:104471.

16. Boppana SB, Fowler KB, Pass RF, et al. Congenital cytomegalovirus infection: association between virus burden in infancy and hearing loss. J Pediatr 2005; 146(6):817–23.

17. Yamaguchi A, Oh-Ishi T, Arai T, et al. Screening for seemingly healthy newborns with congenital cytomegalovirus infection by quantitative real-time polymerase chain reaction using newborn urine: an observational study. BMJ Open 2017; 7(1):e013810.

18. Dahle AJ, Fowler KB, Wright JD, et al. Longitudinal investigation of hearing disorders in children with congenital cytomegalovirus. J Am Acad Audiol 2000;11(5): 283–90.

19. Madden C, Wiley S, Schleiss M, et al. Audiometric, clinical and educational outcomes in a pediatric symptomatic congenital cytomegalovirus (CMV) population with sensorineural hearing loss. Int J Pediatr Otorhinolaryngol 2005;69(9):1191–8.

20. Foulon I, Vleurinck L, Kerkhofs K, et al. Hearing configuration in children with cCMV infection and proposal of a flow chart for hearing evaluation. Int J Audiol 2015;54(10):714–9.

21. Riga M, Korres G, Chouridis P, et al. Congenital cytomegalovirus infection inducing non-congenital sensorineural hearing loss during childhood; a systematic review. Int J Pediatr Otorhinolaryngol 2018;115:156–64.

22. Goderis J, De Leenheer E, Smets K, et al. Hearing loss and congenital CMV infection: a systematic review. Pediatrics 2014;134(5):972–82.

23. Fowler KB, McCollister FP, Dahle AJ, et al. Progressive and fluctuating sensorineural hearing loss in children with asymptomatic congenital cytomegalovirus infection. The J Pediatr 1997;130(4):624–30.

24. Williamson WD, Demmler GJ, Percy AK, et al. Progressive hearing loss in infants with asymptomatic congenital cytomegalovirus infection. Pediatrics 1992;90(6): 862–6.

25. Fowler KB, Dahle AJ, Boppana SB, et al. Newborn hearing screening: will children with hearing loss caused by congenital cytomegalovirus infection be missed? J Pediatr 1999;135(1):60–4.

26. Leruez-Ville M, Vauloup-Fellous C, Couderc S, et al. Prospective identification of congenital cytomegalovirus infection in newborns using real-time polymerase chain reaction assays in dried blood spots. Clin Infect Dis 2011;52(5):575–81.

27. Dollard SC, Dreon M, Hernandez-Alvarado N, et al. Sensitivity of dried blood spot testing for detection of congenital cytomegalovirus infection. JAMA Pediatr 2021; 175(3):e205441.

28. Cannon MJ, Griffiths PD, Aston V, et al. Universal newborn screening for congenital CMV infection: what is the evidence of potential benefit? Rev Med Virol 2014; 24(5):291–307.

29. Grosse SD, Dollard S, Ross DS, et al. Newborn screening for congenital cytomegalovirus: options for hospital-based and public health programs. J Clin Virol 2009;46(Suppl 4):S32–6.

30. Demmler GJ. Screening for congenital cytomegalovirus infection: a tapestry of controversies. J Pediatr 2005;146(2):162–4.

31. Peterson J, Nishimura C, Smith RJH. Genetic testing for congenital bilateral hearing loss in the context of targeted cytomegalovirus screening. Laryngoscope 2020;130(11):2714–8.

32. Ramirez Inscoe JM, Nikolopoulos TP. Cochlear implantation in children deafened by cytomegalovirus: speech perception and speech intelligibility outcomes. Otol Neurotol 2004;25(4):479–82.

33. American Academy of Pediatrics JCoIH. Year 2007 position statement: principles and guidelines for early hearing detection and intervention programs. Pediatrics 2007;120(4):898–921.

34. Royackers L, Christian D, Frans D, et al. Hearing status in children with congenital cytomegalovirus: up-to-6-years audiological follow-up. Int J Pediatr Otorhinolaryngol 2011;75(3):376–82.

35. Lee DJ, Lustig L, Sampson M, et al. Effects of cytomegalovirus (CMV) related deafness on pediatric cochlear implant outcomes. Otolaryngol Head Neck Surg 2005;133(6):900–5.

36. Iwasaki S, Nakanishi H, Misawa K, et al. Cochlear implant in children with asymptomatic congenital cytomegalovirus infection. Audiol Neurootol 2009;14(3):146–52.

37. Yoshida H, Takahashi H, Kanda Y, et al. Long-term outcomes of cochlear implantation in children with congenital cytomegalovirus infection. Otol Neurotol 2017;38(7):e190–4.

38. Ciorba A, Bovo R, Trevisi P, et al. Rehabilitation and outcome of severe profound deafness in a group of 16 infants affected by congenital cytomegalovirus infection. Eur Arch Otorhinolaryngol 2009;266(10):1539–46.

39. Philips B, Maes LK, Keppler H, et al. Cochlear implants in children deafened by congenital cytomegalovirus and matched connexin 26 peers. Int J Pediatr Otorhinolaryngol 2014;78(3):410–5.

40. Hoff S, Ryan M, Thomas D, et al. Safety and effectiveness of cochlear implantation of young children, including those with complicating conditions. Otol Neurotol 2019;40(4):454–63.

41. Yoshida H, Kanda Y, Takahashi H, et al. Cochlear implantation in children with congenital cytomegalovirus infection. Otol Neurotol 2009;30(6):725–30.

42. Young N, Weil C, Tournis E. Redefining cochlear implant benefits to appropriately include children with additional disabilities. In: Young N, Kirk K, editors. Pediatric cochlear implantation. New York, NY: Springer-Verlag; 2016. p. 213–26.

43. Wiley S, Jahnke M, Meinzen-Derr J, et al. Perceived qualitative benefits of cochlear implants in children with multi-handicaps. Int J Pediatr Otorhinolaryngol 2005;69(6):791–8.

44. Waltzman S, Scalchunes V, Cohen N. Performance of multiply handicapped children using cochlear implants. Am J Otolaryngol 2000;21(3):329–35.

45. Coats DK, Demmler GJ, Paysse EA, et al. Ophthalmologic findings in children with congenital cytomegalovirus infection. J AAPOS 2000;4(2):110–6.

46. Whitley RJ, Cloud G, Gruber W, et al. Ganciclovir treatment of symptomatic congenital cytomegalovirus infection: results of a phase II study. National Institute of Allergy and Infectious Diseases Collaborative Antiviral Study Group. J Infect Dis 1997;175(5):1080–6.
47. Kimberlin DW, Lin C-Y, Sánchez PJ, et al. Effect of ganciclovir therapy on hearing in symptomatic congenital cytomegalovirus disease involving the central nervous system: a randomized, controlled trial. J Pediatr 2003;143(1):16–25.
48. Oliver SE, Cloud GA, Sanchez PJ, et al. Neurodevelopmental outcomes following ganciclovir therapy in symptomatic congenital cytomegalovirus infections involving the central nervous system. J Clin Virol 2009;46(Suppl 4):S22–6.
49. Acosta EP, Brundage RC, King JR, et al. Ganciclovir population pharmacokinetics in neonates following intravenous administration of ganciclovir and oral administration of a liquid valganciclovir formulation. Clin Pharmacol Ther 2007; 81(6):867–72.
50. Kimberlin DW, Acosta EP, Sanchez PJ, et al. Pharmacokinetic and pharmacodynamic assessment of oral valganciclovir in the treatment of symptomatic congenital cytomegalovirus disease. J Infect Dis 2008;197(6):836–45.
51. Kimberlin DW, Jester PM, Sanchez PJ, et al. Valganciclovir for symptomatic congenital cytomegalovirus disease. N Engl J Med 2015;372(10):933–43.
52. Rawlinson WD, Boppana SB, Fowler KB, et al. Congenital cytomegalovirus infection in pregnancy and the neonate: consensus recommendations for prevention, diagnosis, and therapy. The Lancet Infect Dis 2017;17(6):e177–88.
53. Dorfman L, Amir J, Attias J, et al. Treatment of congenital cytomegalovirus beyond the neonatal period: an observational study. Eur J Pediatr 2020;179(5): 807–12.
54. del Rosal T, Baquero-Artigao F, Blazquez D, et al. Treatment of symptomatic congenital cytomegalovirus infection beyond the neonatal period. J Clin Virol 2012;55(1):72–4.

Pediatric Hearing Loss Guidelines and Consensus Statements—Where Do We Stand?

Samantha J. Gustafson, AuD, PhD[a],*, Nicole E. Corbin, AuD, PhD[b]

KEYWORDS

- Hearing loss • Children • Guidelines • Screening • Diagnosis • Intervention

KEY POINTS

- Infants should be screened for hearing loss by 1 month of age, diagnosed by 3 months, and enrolled in intervention services by 6 months (1-3-6 goal). For systems currently meeting the 1-3-6 goal, a 1-2-3 goal is recommended.
- Infants who pass the newborn hearing screening and possess or develop any of the 12 known risk factors for childhood hearing loss should be monitored regularly for indicators of congenital, delayed-onset, or progressive hearing loss.
- Once a hearing loss is diagnosed, the otolaryngologist should partner with the medical home provider and audiologist to facilitate coordinated and comprehensive care, including the referral to early intervention and fitting of amplification.

Evidence-based practice (EBP), or evidence-based medicine, involves the integration of scientific evidence, clinical expertise, and patient/family values to provide optimal patient care.[1] Given the current rate of technological development and scientific discovery, clinical practice guidelines (CPGs) and consensus or position statements are essential tools for health care professionals providing EBP.[2] A CPG is functionally the same as a consensus or position statement and is the preferred term used in this article. CPGs describe how members of a given profession should adhere to a standard of practice, ensuring that patients receive consistent, high-quality care regardless of setting or provider.[2] The purpose of this article is to review the current state of CPGs as they relate to children with hearing loss.

SCREENING FOR PEDIATRIC HEARING LOSS

Many CPGs have been developed to identify children who have or are at risk for developing hearing loss. This is in response to overwhelming evidence that children with

[a] University of Utah, 390 South 1530 East, BEH-S 1201, Salt Lake City, UT 84112, USA;
[b] University of Pittsburgh, 6035 Forbes Tower, Pittsburgh, PA 15260, USA
* Corresponding author.
E-mail address: samantha.gustafson@utah.edu

Otolaryngol Clin N Am 54 (2021) 1129–1142
https://doi.org/10.1016/j.otc.2021.07.003   oto.theclinics.com

hearing loss who receive early identification and intervention achieve better academic, cognitive, communication, language, and social-emotional outcomes than those who do not.[3,4] Given that hearing loss is one of the most prevalent developmental disabilities at birth,[5] the first entry point for identification and intervention of childhood hearing loss is through newborn hearing screening (NBHS).

Newborn Screening via Early Hearing Detection and Intervention Systems

The Joint Committee on Infant Hearing (JCIH) publishes CPGs for the development and implementation of universal NBHS programs, which now are designated early hearing detection and intervention (EHDI) systems. The use of the term EHDI is preferred, because it underscores the importance of NBHS being tied to an entire system that includes the medical home, a tracking and surveillance process, a method for monitoring system efficacy, audiologic diagnosis, and appropriate intervention services in partnership with the family[6] (**Box 1**). The overall goal of EHDI is to identify infants with hearing loss as early as possible to optimize overall development through early and consistent access to language and intervention services. Components of successful EHDI systems are shown in **Box 2** and a flowchart detailing the preferred progression of EHDI activities is provided in **Fig. 1**. Generally, EHDI recommends that infants are screened for hearing loss by 1 month of age, receive confirmation of hearing status by 3 months of age, and begin intervention services (if indicated) by 6 months of age (1-3-6 goals). JCIH recently suggested that EHDI systems currently meeting 1-3-6 goals consider establishing 1-2-3 goals (audiologic screening by 1 month, audiologic diagnosis by 2 months, and intervention initiated by 3 months). The rationale for establishing a 1-2-3 timeline includes providing infants even earlier access to language and reducing the likelihood of administering sedation to complete audiologic testing in infancy. The 1-2-3 timeline may not be feasible for very preterm infants who could remain in the neonatal intensive care unit through the third month of life. For those infants, JCIH recommends a diagnostic audiologic evaluation prior to discharge and direct referral to audiologic follow-up and early intervention services as appropriate.

The preferred method for conducting NBHS in the well-baby nursery is either automated auditory brainstem response (AABR) or otoacoustic emissions (OAEs).[9] For infants in the well-baby nursery who fail the initial NBHS, the second screening (eg, rescreen) should be conducted on both ears using either method; however, it is preferred that infants who fail the initial screening conducted by AABR are rescreened using AABR.[9] JCIH recommends initial and rescreening protocols in neonatal intensive care units be conducted solely with AABR in the hospital or by a pediatric audiologist in an outpatient setting.[9]

JCIH recognizes that NBHS protocols do not identify all children with hearing loss given the reasons listed in **Table 1**. Because not all childhood hearing loss is present

---

Box 1
Importance of advocating for EHDI funding

Federal funding for EHDI systems currently comes from the Department of Health and Human Services.[7] At the state and territory levels, funding for EHDI systems varies according to a variety of factors including Medicaid, Title V funding, general revenues, and procured grants. For these reasons, public and professional advocacy for EHDI at the federal, state, and territory levels is essential for the continuation and improvement of EHDI systems. As of March 2021, all 50 states and the District of Columbia have EHDI systems, with 43 states containing legislation describing minimum standards for their EHDI system.

Box 2
Components of successful early hearing detection and intervention systems

- All infants undergo NBHS by 1 month of age, prior to discharge from the birthing hospital
  - Infants who fail NBHS in either ear are scheduled for an appointment for outpatient rescreening or audiologic evaluation at the time of hospital discharge.
  - Alternate contact information for a family is obtained.
  - Regardless of NBHS result, the communication development of all infants and children is monitored by professionals with appropriate training and within the medical home according to the AAP Periodicity Schedule.[8]

- All infants who fail the NBHS have an audiologic diagnostic assessment by 3 months of age.
  - For infants who are diagnosed with hearing loss, the following should occur concurrently or immediately after diagnosis:
    - Otologic evaluation
    - Referral to an appropriate interdisciplinary early intervention system through a simplified, coordinated point of entry
      - This referral is made by a professional knowledgeable about the needs and requirements of children with hearing loss.

- All infants who are diagnosed with hearing loss begin early intervention services as soon as possible after audiologic diagnosis and no later than 6 months of age.
  - The early intervention approach documented in an Individualized Family Service Plan honors the family's preferences and goals for their child.
    - The approach builds on the strengths, informed choices, language traditions, and cultural beliefs of the family.
  - The child and family have *immediate* access to hearing aid technology through their audiologist.
  - The child and family have access to cochlear implants, hearing assistive technologies, and visual alerting and informational devices.
  - The family has access to
    - Information about all resources and programs for intervention
    - Support and counseling about the child's educational and communication needs

- Individualized, family-centered care

- Informed and shared decision making

- EBP

- Guarantee of family rights and privacy

- Family consent following state and federal guidelines

- Information systems that facilitate exchange of electronic health information with clinical electronic health records and population-based information systems

---

at birth, infants who pass the NBHS and possess or develop any of the 12 known risk factors for early childhood hearing loss listed in **Table 2** should be monitored as indicated.

Continued Screening for Childhood Hearing Loss

The prevalence of hearing loss increases by the time children enter school.[11,12] As of March 2021, there is no CPG or federal mandate regarding universal hearing screening after the newborn period.[10] Some states mandate school-based screenings whereas others do not. Therefore, all infants and children, regardless of presence or absence of risk factors, should receive ongoing surveillance of communication development.[8,9,13] It is the otolaryngologist's responsibility to evaluate all infants and children on their caseload for the risk factors listed in **Table 2**. For specific recommendations regarding the otolaryngologic work-up of hearing loss in children, please reference Sampat

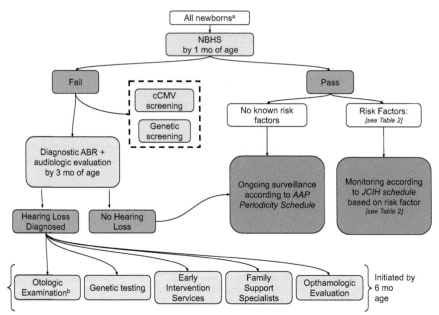

Fig. 1. Preferred progress of EHDI activities outlined by JCIH.[9] Green shading represents stages of assessment, with possible results shown in blue. The dashed box represents assessments not yet used in widespread clinical practice. Red shading represents patient management. [a]JCIH recognizes that this timeline may not be feasible for preterm infants who require prolonged hospitalization in the Neonatal Intensive Care Unit. [b]Sometimes the otologic examination occurs in conjunction with the diagnostic ABR + audiologic evaluation. (*Data from* Year 2019 Position Statement: Principles and Guidelines for Early Hearing Detection and Intervention Programs. Journal of Early Hearing Detection and Intervention. 2019;4(2):1-44. https://doi.org/10.15142/FPTK-B748.)

Sindhar and Judith E.C. Lieu's article, "Overview of Medical Evaluation of Unilateral & Bilateral Hearing Loss in Children," in this issue.

Special Considerations

Cytomegalovirus

Cytomegalovirus is the leading cause of congenital infection, occurring in 0.2% to 2% of live births worldwide. The 2019 JCIH guidelines acknowledge that congenital cytomegalovirus (cCMV) plays a larger role in childhood hearing loss than previously thought, with 10% to 15% of infants with cCMV developing sensorineural hearing loss.[9] A 2015 International Congenital Cytomegalovirus Recommendations Group suggested that universal screening for cCMV in all newborns should be considered but fell short of providing a recommendation for universal screening, citing the need for prospective studies and cost-effectiveness studies prior to a recommendation.[14] In 2019, the Newborn Hearing Screening Working Group of the National Coordinating Center for the Regional Genetics Networks recommended that universal cCMV screening, along with limited genetic testing, be integrated into the current NBHS program.[15] Although the development of an appropriate and relatively inexpensive screening has been a priority research topic for nearly 2 decades,[16] nationwide screening for cCMV does not exist as of March 2021. In line with the International Pediatric Otolaryngology Group recommendations,[17] several states have implemented

Table 1 Reasons children with hearing loss may not be identified by newborn hearing screening[9,10]	
Early Hearing Detection and Intervention Outcome	**Potential Reason for Undiagnosed Childhood Hearing Loss**
Child passed NBHS	No hearing loss present at time of NBHS (eg, delayed onset of hearing loss)
	Hearing loss present but not detected by NBHS due to limitations of sensitivity and specificity of the NBHS protocol
	Hearing loss present but not detected by NBHS (eg, mild hearing loss or auditory neuropathy spectrum disorder)
	Progressive or fluctuating hearing loss
	Screening equipment or personnel error
Child missed NBHS	Parent refusal
	Not birthed in a hospital
	Hospital discharge or transfer prior to completion of NBHS
	Rescreen never completed after initial fail result
Child lost to follow-up or documentation	NBHS completed in another state
	Miscommunication or lack of communication regarding NBHS result to family, medical and health care providers, hospitals, and/or state EHDI system
	Lack of or poor documentation of NBHS result, diagnostic assessment, or referral to early intervention services
	Parent or physician misunderstanding of or lack of commitment to follow-up when indicated (eg, fail result or presence of risk factor[s] listed in **Table 2**)
	Lack of skilled pediatric audiology services near the family's home
	Family challenges with transportation to follow-up appointments or services
	Infant does not have established care with a primary care provider or medical home
	Parent does not consent to diagnostic evaluation or early intervention services
	Unable to make contact with family

Data from Year 2019 Position Statement: Principles and Guidelines for Early Hearing Detection and Intervention Programs. Journal of Early Hearing Detection and Intervention. 2019;4(2):1-44. https://doi.org/10.15142/FPTK-B748, Hall J. Effective And Efficient Pre-School Hearing Screening: Essential For Successful EHDI. Journal of Early Hearing Detection and Intervention. 2016;1(1):2-12. https://doi.org/10.15142/T3XW2F.

targeted cCMV screening—testing children who fail NBHS.[18] Early findings with targeted cCMV screening show that, although sensitivity was not as high as universal cCMV screening, more than two-thirds of symptomatic cCMV cases could be identified with this approach.[19]

Zika virus
The Zika virus is a mosquito-borne infection that can be passed from a pregnant woman to a developing fetus. Congenital Zika syndrome (CZS) causes birth defects,

Table 2
Twelve risk factors for early childhood hearing loss: guidelines for infants who pass newborn hearing screening

Risk Factor Classification	Recommended Diagnostic Follow-up	Monitoring Frequency
Perinatal		
Family history[a] of early, progressive, or delayed-onset permanent childhood hearing loss	By 9 mo	Based on etiology of family hearing loss and caregiver concern
Neonatal intensive care >5 d	By 9 mo	As per concerns of ongoing surveillance of communication development
Hyperbilirubinemia with exchange transfusion regardless of length of stay	By 9 mo	
Aminoglycoside administration >5 d or <5 d if toxic blood levels are identified or a genetic susceptibility is known	By 9 mo	
Asphyxia or hypoxic ischemic encephalopathy	By 9 mo	
Extracorporeal membrane oxygenation	No later than 3 mo after occurrence	Every 12 mo to school age or at shorter intervals based on parent/provider concerns
In utero infections, such as herpes, rubella, syphilis, and toxoplasmosis	By 9 mo	As per concerns of ongoing surveillance
In utero infection with cytomegalovirus	No later than 3 mo after occurrence	Every 12 mo to age 3 or at shorter intervals based on parent/provider concerns
Mother positive for Zika virus	Standard	As per AAP Periodicity Schedule [8]
• Infant with no laboratory evidence and no clinical findings	AABR by 1 mo	ABR by 4–6 mo or visual reinforcement audiometry by 9 mo
• Infant with laboratory evidence of Zika and no clinical findings	AABR by 1 mo	ABR by 4–6 mo
• Infant with laboratory evidence of Zika and no clinical findings		Monitor as per AAP Periodicity Schedule [8]
Certain birth conditions or findings • Craniofacial malformations including microtia/atresia, ear dysplasia, oral facial clefting, white forelock, and microphthalmia • Congenital microcephaly, congenital or acquired hydrocephalus • Temporal bone abnormalities	By 9 mo	As per concerns of ongoing surveillance of communication development

More than 400 syndromes have been identified with atypical hearing thresholds. Visit https://hereditaryhearingloss.org/for more information.	By 9 mo	According to natural history of syndrome or concerns
Perinatal or postnatal		
Culture-positive infections associated with sensorineural hearing loss, including confirmed bacterial and viral (especially herpes viruses and varicella) meningitis or encephalitis	No later than 3 mo after occurrence	Every 12 mo to school age or at shorter intervals based on parent/provider concerns
Events associated with hearing loss • Significant head trauma, especially basal skull/temporal bone fractures • Chemotherapy	No later than 3 mo after occurrence	According to findings and/or continued concerns
Caregiver concern regarding hearing, speech, language, developmental delay, and/or developmental regression	Immediate referral	According to findings and/or continued concern

[a] Infants at increased risk of delayed onset or progressive hearing loss.

Adapted from "Year 2019 Position Statement: Principles and Guidelines for Early Hearing Detection and Intervention Programs," by Journal of Early Hearing Detection and Intervention, 4(2), p. 19 (https://digitalcommons.usu.edu/jehdi/vol4/iss2/1). CC BY-NC.

such as microcephaly, decreased brain tissue, and vision and hearing impairment. Approximately 7% of infants with CZS have sensorineural hearing loss.[20] Although the Zika virus is not an epidemic in the United States, CZS still is a concern in Central and South American countries, where the Zika virus remains a threat. For the first time, JCIH has included the Zika virus in its list of risk factors for hearing loss. JCIH and Centers for Disease Control and Prevention (CDC) recommendations for testing the hearing of infants with Zika virus are shown in **Box 3**. Although the primary concern for Zika virus infections is CZS, children infected with Zika beyond the neonatal period are at risk for Guillain-Barré syndrome and transient sensorineural hearing loss.

DIAGNOSING PEDIATRIC HEARING LOSS

Audiologic diagnosis of hearing loss should be completed no later than 2 months to 3 months of age by an audiologist with the specific skills, knowledge, and access to equipment required for infant and early childhood diagnostic evaluations. Pediatric audiologists can be found through a roster maintained by the American Board of Audiology or through the EHDI Pediatric Audiology Links to Service.[21] Testing included in an audiologic diagnostic appointment is listed in **Table 3**. The auditory brainstem response (ABR) is not a test of hearing, but a measure of an electrophysiologic response to auditory stimuli. To confirm a child's hearing (perception), a behavioral evaluation should be conducted as soon as the child is developmentally capable of providing reliable responses (approximately 6 months of age).

The Role of the Medical Home

Because the rate of childhood hearing loss increases from 1.2/1000 in newborns to 3/1000 in early school age,[22] all children, regardless of NBHS result, should receive surveillance of speech and language milestones and auditory development in the medical home beginning at 2 months of age.[8] Ongoing screening allows for children with delayed-onset or progressive hearing loss or those who might have been missed by NBHS (eg, mild hearing loss) to receive timely intervention. Once diagnosed, the medical home provider should refer the child with hearing loss to an otolaryngologist, clinical geneticist, genetic counselor, audiologist, speech-language pathologist, early hearing intervention provider, and family support specialist. This team of professionals should collaborate with the family in informed decision making for their child.[23] This care is ideally found at a multidisciplinary care center; however, in some areas, families

---

Box 3
Joint Committee on Infant Hearing and Centers for Disease Control and Prevention share recommendations for audiologic testing of infants with Zika virus

- Infants with laboratory-confirmed Zika—regardless of symptoms—should receive an automated ABR by 1 month even if they passed a NBHS with OAEs.

- Infants with laboratory-confirmed Zika with clinical symptoms also should receive a diagnostic ABR by 4 months to 6 months or testing using visual response audiometry by 9 months of age.

- Infants with laboratory-confirmed Zika with no clinical symptoms should receive a diagnostic ABR by 4 months to 6 months.

- From thereafter, the AAP 2017 schedule of testing for infants with risk factors[8] should be followed for all infants with Zika virus.

Table 3 Key aspects of audiologic assessment for infants and young children	
ABR	Gold standard test for infants and children who cannot complete behavioral audiologic assessment; provides information necessary to diagnose the type, degree, and configuration of hearing loss
Tympanometry or wideband reflectance	Measures of middle ear function
Acoustic reflexes	Test of middle ear function and integrity of auditory brainstem pathways
OAEs	Assessment of integrity of the outer hair cells of the cochlea Critical for the differential diagnosis of auditory neuropathy spectrum disorder and sensorineural hearing loss
Behavioral assessment of hearing	Gold standard test for infants and children who can provide reliable and valid responses

might need to seek services from individual providers. Finally, because the otolaryngologist's evaluation includes a comprehensive history to identify risk factors for and findings associated with congenital or delayed-onset childhood hearing loss (see Cynthia Casson Morton's article, "Genetics of Childhood Hearing Loss," in this issue), the otolaryngologist should partner with the medical home provider and audiologist to facilitate coordinated and comprehensive care.

Genetic Screening

It is estimated that up to 60% of congenital and early-onset hearing loss is caused by genetic factors.[24,25] In conjunction with the American College of Medical Genetics and Genomics, JCIH recommends that all infants and children with confirmed hearing loss be offered genetics evaluation and counseling.[9,26] Results of genetic testing can be valuable for families of children with hearing loss, providing answers to 2 common questions: (1) "What caused my child's hearing loss?" and (2) "Will their hearing loss change over time?" In addition to information about the etiology and prognosis for progression, genetic evaluation can uncover disorders associated with the hearing loss (eg, renal, vision, and cardiac) and explain the likelihood of recurrence of hearing loss in future offspring.

INTERVENTION AND MANAGEMENT OF PEDIATRIC HEARING LOSS

Together with the American Academy of Pediatrics (AAP) and CDC, JCIH recommends that, at the time of hearing loss diagnosis, children should be referred for medical and otologic evaluations to the state EHDI program and to the state Part C early intervention program.[8,13,27,28] The purposes of the medical and otologic evaluations are to identify any conditions related to the hearing loss, provide medical/surgical recommendations and treatments, refer the child for ancillary services, and engage the family in informed decision making for their child[23] (**Box 4**). Once medical clearance is obtained, children with hearing loss should be fitted with hearing aids by an audiologist with expertise, skills, and knowledge in pediatric audiology.[30] JCIH recommends fitting of amplification as soon as possible following the diagnosis of hearing loss. Children with sensorineural hearing loss will be fitted with traditional air conduction hearing aids, which might be contraindicated for some children (eg, draining ears and microtia). In these cases, it is important that

---

Box 4
Medical clearance for amplification

For families who have chosen listening and spoken language as the communication goal for their child, medical clearance to obtain hearing aids is included as part of these medical recommendations. Specifically, the Food and Drug Administration requires a written statement from a licensed physician declaring that a medical evaluation has determined the patient to be a candidate for hearing aids.[29] As of 2020, federal law allows a fully informed adult to sign a waiver declining the medical evaluation—this option is not permitted for children. Importantly, medical clearance for hearing aid fitting should not be delayed until other medical examinations are completed or a diagnosis of etiology made.

---

infants and young children with conductive hearing loss be fitted with bone conduction hearing devices on a softband until they are considered implant candidates at age 5 years. Once fitted, the child receives regular surveillance of hearing status and ongoing validation of amplification fitting. A child's referral to early intervention should not be deferred until hearing aid fitting; referral should occur within 48 hours of hearing loss diagnosis.[31]

For children who fail to make expected progress with appropriately fitted amplification, cochlear implantation evaluation should be offered, especially if parental goals for their child include improved hearing and understanding and the use of spoken language. The cochlear implant evaluation process should be conducted by a team consisting of audiologists, otolaryngologists, medical home providers, early intervention specialists, and the family. Cochlear implantation is currently approved by the US Food and Drug Administration for children 9 months of age and older, and clinical trials to reduce age further are underway. Age at implant and audiologic candidacy for cochlear implantation is expanding (see Rene H. Gifford's article, "Expanded Criteria for Cochlear Implantation of Children with Bilateral Sensorineural Hearing Loss," in this issue). The American Academy of Otolaryngology-Head and Neck Surgery (AAO-HNS) now considers cochlear implantation (unilateral and bilateral) an appropriate treatment of children, including infants between 6 months and 12 months of age with severe to profound hearing loss having failed a trial with appropriately fitted hearing aids. Children aged 12 months and older with more residual hearing (pure tone average between 65 dB and 85 dB) might be candidates if aided auditory skill development and speech and language progress indicate persistent or widening gap in age-appropriate skills.[32]

Chronic Middle Ear Conditions

Otitis media with effusion (OME) typically resolves within 3 months, but 30% to 40% of children have repeated episodes of OME, with 5% to 10% of episodes lasting more than 1 year.[33,34] This middle ear fluid can be associated with conductive hearing loss, placing some children at risk for developmental difficulties. The AAO-HNS CPG for OME[35] identifies 7 risk factors for developmental difficulties in children with OME (**Box 5**).

Recommendations for management of OME in children without permanent hearing loss vary widely. Recent guidelines pertaining to OME management are as follows.

- The AAO-HNS recommends that a child with persistent OME and no known risk factors for permanent hearing loss be managed with watchful waiting for 3 months from the date of effusion onset (if known) or from date of diagnosis if onset is unknown. If OME persists for greater than or equal to 3 months or

---

Box 5
Risk factors for developmental difficulties associated with childhood otitis media with effusion, as specified by the American Academy of Otolaryngology-Head and Neck Surgery clinical practice guidelines

Permanent hearing loss independent of OME

Suspected or confirmed speech and language delay or disorder

Autistic spectrum disorder

Syndromes or craniofacial disorders that include cognitive, speech, or language delays

Blindness or uncorrectable visual impairment

Cleft palate

Developmental delay

---

if OME of any duration is present in an at-risk child, a full audiologic evaluation should be recommended. AAO-HNS also recommends that children with chronic OME be evaluated in 3-month to 6-month intervals until OME is resolved, significant hearing loss is identified, or structural abnormalities are suspected. Note that the definition of *significant hearing loss* intentionally was not defined in this guideline.

- JCIH takes a more conservative approach by recommending that a child with OME persisting for greater than or equal to 6 months should be referred for early intervention services to ensure adequate auditory access.[31]
- Perhaps the most conservative approach to chronic OME is taken by the International Pediatric Otolaryngology Group, which recommends that children with persistent OME within the first few months of life receive myringotomy and tubes with a follow-up ABR if OME still is present at 6 months of age.[17]

Guidelines for management of OME were developed for children with normal hearing sensitivity. More aggressive management of OME in children with permanent hearing loss should be considered. Quickly resolving OME in children with permanent hearing loss is essential for the accurate initial diagnosis of degree of loss and to optimize benefits from amplification. Furthermore, because some infants and children do not tolerate hearing devices when OME is present, speedy resolution of OME can aid in consistent use of amplification.

Ototoxicity-induced hearing loss

Approximately half of pediatric survivors of cancer develop hearing loss as a result of ototoxicity from treatment with platinum-base compounds and/or radiation of the head or brain.[36,37] Because ototoxicity-induced hearing loss often affects the high frequencies and presents with tinnitus, audiologic surveillance is recommended for pediatric survivors of cancer treated with head or brain radiotherapy or with cisplatin, with or without high-dose carboplatin (**Box 6**).[38] This recommendation holds true regardless of cotreatment with otoprotective agents.[38,39] Ideally, a baseline audiologic evaluation establishes hearing thresholds prior to the initiation of oncologic treatment. Otolaryngologists should communicate directly with oncology regarding treatment and with audiology regarding hearing surveillance. Refer to Peter S. Steyger's article, "Mechanisms of Ototoxicity & Otoprotection," in this issue for additional information about ototoxicity and otoprotection.

Box 6
Monitoring ototoxicity-induced hearing loss

Audiologic surveillance should begin prior to the end of oncologic treatment. When treatment begins at less than 6 years of age, audiologic surveillance should continue, at minimum, annually. For children who begin treatment at 6 years and 12 years of age, audiologic surveillance should occur every other year. When treatment begins at greater than 12 years of age, audiologic surveillance should occur every 5 years.[38] Beyond these recommendations, there is no consensus regarding how long ototoxicity-induced hearing loss monitoring should continue past treatment.

SUMMARY

The implementation of CPGs that guide screening, diagnosis, and management of hearing loss in children has resulted in improved outcomes for children with hearing loss. Not all infants and children, however, with hearing loss receive timely diagnosis and intervention. As a result, it is critical that the otolaryngologist evaluate all infants and children for risk factors for hearing loss, regardless of NBHS result, and make prompt referrals when indicated. Although not yet covered in CPGs, otolaryngologists should also consider the impact of cerumen, noise exposure, and potentially COVID-19 infection on children's hearing status.

CLINICS CARE POINTS

---

1. NBHS testing method
   For infants in the well-baby nursery who fail the initial NBHS, it is preferred that the second screening be conducted on both ears using AABR. Neonatal intensive care unit initial and rescreening protocols should be conducted solely with AABR.

2. Risk factor monitoring
   Risk factor assessment is important when evaluating children who passed NBHS. Those at risk for postnatal onset of hearing loss (see **Table 2**) should be referred for audiologic evaluation and monitoring. Of special consideration are children with positive neonatal viral cultures or microcephaly and other findings concerning cCMV or Zika.

3. Otitis media management
   Guidelines for management of otitis media were developed for children with normal hearing sensitivity who are not at risk for language delay. Children with permanent hearing loss could benefit from timelier placement of myringotomy tubes than indicated in these guidelines.

4. Cochlear implantation evaluation
   Infants with bilateral severe profound hearing loss and young children with moderate to severe loss not progressing despite amplification would benefit from referral to candidacy evaluation by a pediatric cochlear implant program.

DISCLOSURE

The authors have no commercial or financial conflicts of interest to disclose.

REFERENCES

1. Sackett DL, Rosenberg WM, Gray JA, et al. Evidence based medicine: what it is and what it isn't. BMJ 1996;312(7023):71–2.
2. Coverstone J. The need for standards in audiology. Hearing Rev 2019; 26(3):24–9.

3. Moeller MP. Early intervention and language development in children who are deaf and hard of hearing. Pediatrics 2000;106(3):E43.
4. Yoshinaga-Itano C, Sedey AL, Coulter DK, et al. Language of early- and later-identified children with hearing loss. Pediatrics 1998;102(5):1161–71.
5. CDC. Data and Statistics About Hearing Loss in Children | CDC. Centers for Disease Control and Prevention. 2020. Available at: https://www.cdc.gov/ncbddd/hearingloss/data.html. Accessed March 29, 2021.
6. White KR. Chapter 1: the evolution of EHDI: from concept to standard of care. In: The NCHAM EBook. National Center for Hearing Assessment and Management Utah State University; 2021. p. 32. Available at: http://www.infanthearing.org/ehdi-ebook/index.html. Accessed February 1, 2021.
7. Early hearing detection and intervention act. 2017;42 C.F.R. § 280g-1(a).
8. Medicine C on P and A, Workgroup BFPS. 2017 recommendations for preventive pediatric health care. Pediatrics 2017;139(4):e20170254.
9. Year 2019 position statement: principles and guidelines for early hearing detection and intervention programs. J Early Hear Detect Interv 2019;4(2):1–44.
10. Hall J. Effective and efficient pre-school hearing screening: essential for successful EHDI. J Early Hear Detect Interv 2016;1(1):2–12.
11. Fortnum HM, Summerfield AQ, Marshall DH, et al. Prevalence of permanent childhood hearing impairment in the United Kingdom and implications for universal neonatal hearing screening: questionnaire based ascertainment study. BMJ 2001;323(7312):536–40.
12. Shargorodsky J, Curhan SG, Curhan GC, et al. Change in prevalence of hearing loss in US adolescents. JAMA 2010;304(7):772–8.
13. American Academy of Pediatrics. Reducing loss to follow-up/document in newborn hearing screening: guidelines for medical home providers 2014. Available at: http://www.aap.org/en-us/Documents/ehdi_ltfdguidelines.pdf.
14. Rawlinson WD, Boppana SB, Fowler KB, et al. Congenital cytomegalovirus infection in pregnancy and the neonate: consensus recommendations for prevention, diagnosis, and therapy. Lancet Infect Dis 2017;17(6):e177–88.
15. Shearer AE, Shen J, Amr S, et al. A proposal for comprehensive newborn hearing screening to improve identification of deaf and hard-of-hearing children. Genet Med 2019;21(11):2614–30.
16. NIDCD workshop on congenital cytomegalovirus infection and hearing loss. NIDCD. Available at: https://www.nidcd.nih.gov/research/workshops/congenital-cytomegalovirus-infection-and-hearing-loss/2002. Accessed February 1, 2021.
17. Liming BJ, Carter J, Cheng A, et al. International Pediatric Otolaryngology Group (IPOG) consensus recommendations: hearing loss in the pediatric patient. Int J Pediatr Otorhinolaryngol 2016;90:251–8.
18. Haller T, Shoup A, Park A. Should hearing targeted screening for congenital cytomegalovirus infection be implemented? Int J Pediatr otorhinolaryngol 2020;110055.
19. McCrary H, Shi K, Newberry IC, et al. Outcomes from an expanded targeted early cytomegalovirus testing program. J Pediatr Infect Dis 2020;15(04):189–94.
20. Leal MC, Muniz L, Ferreira T, et al. Hearing loss in infants with microcephaly and evidence of congenital zika virus infection — Brazil, November 2015–May 2016. MMWR Morb Mortal Wkly Rep 2016;65:917–9.
21. EHDI-PALS. Available at: https://www.ehdi-pals.org/default.aspx. Accessed February 8, 2021.

22. Watkin P, Baldwin M. The longitudinal follow up of a universal neonatal hearing screen: the implications for confirming deafness in childhood. Int J Audiol 2012;51(7):519–28.

23. Prosser JD, Cohen AP, Greinwald JH. Diagnostic evaluation of children with sensorineural hearing loss. Otolaryngol Clin North Am 2015;48(6):975–82.

24. Mitchell RE, Karchmer M. Chasing the mythical ten percent: Parental hearing status of deaf and hard of hearing students in the United States. Sign Lang Stud 2004;4(2):138–63.

25. Marazita ML, Ploughman LM, Rawlings B, et al. Genetic epidemiological studies of early-onset deafness in the US school-age population. Am J Med Genet 1993; 46(5):486–91.

26. Alford RL, Arnos KS, Fox M, et al. American College of Medical Genetics and Genomics guideline for the clinical evaluation and etiologic diagnosis of hearing loss. Genet Med 2014;16(4):347.

27. American Academy of Pediatrics. Guidelines for rescreening in the medical home following a "do not pass" newborn hearing screening 2014. Available at: https://tinyurl.com/y5p2k953.

28. Centers for Disease Control and Prevention. Information about early hearing detection and intervention (EHDI) state programs. Hearing loss in children 2016. Available at: http://www.cdc.gov/ncbddd/hearingloss/ehdi-programs.html.

29. Hearing aid devices; professional and patient labeling. 2020;21 C.F.R. § 801.420.

30. Bagatto M, Moodie S, Brown C, et al. Prescribing and verifying hearing aids applying the American Academy of Audiology pediatric amplification guideline: protocols and outcomes from the Ontario infant hearing program. J Am Acad Audiol 2016;27(3):188–203.

31. Muse C, Harrison J, Yoshinaga-Itano C, et al. Supplement to the JCIH 2007 position statement: Principles and guidelines for early intervention after confirmation that a child is deaf or hard of hearing. Pediatrics 2013;131(4):e1324–49.

32. American Academy of Otolaryngology-Head and Neck Surgery. Shelton (CT): Position statement: cochlear implants. 2020. Available at: https://www.entnet.org/content/position-statement-cochlear-implants. Accessed February 15, 2021.

33. Rosenfeld RM. A Parent's guide to ear tubes. PMPH-USA; 2005.

34. Williamson IG, Dunleavey J, Bain J, et al. The natural history of otitis media with effusion–a three-year study of the incidence and prevalence of abnormal tympanograms in four South West Hampshire infant and first schools. J Laryngol Otol 1994;108(11):930–4.

35. Rosenfeld RM, Shin JJ, Schwartz SR, et al. Clinical practice guideline: otitis media with effusion (update). Otolaryngol Head Neck Surg 2016;154(1_suppl):S1–41.

36. Knight KRG, Kraemer DF, Neuwelt EA. Ototoxicity in children receiving platinum chemotherapy: underestimating a commonly occurring toxicity that may influence academic and social development. J Clin Oncol 2005;23(34):8588–96.

37. Bass JK, Hua C-H, Huang J, et al. Hearing loss in patients who received cranial radiation therapy for childhood cancer. J Clin Oncol 2016;34(11):1248–55.

38. Clemens E, van den Heuvel-Eibrink MM, Mulder RL, et al. Recommendations for ototoxicity surveillance for childhood, adolescent, and young adult cancer survivors: a report from the International late effects of Childhood Cancer Guideline Harmonization Group in collaboration with the PanCare Consortium. Lancet Oncol 2019;20(1):e29–41.

39. Freyer DR, Brock PR, Chang KW, et al. Prevention of cisplatin-induced ototoxicity in children and adolescents with cancer: a clinical practice guideline. Lancet Child Adolesc Health 2020;4(2):141–50.

Clinical Test Batteries to Diagnose Hearing Loss in Infants and Children
The Cross-Check Principle

Joy Ringger, AuD[a],*, Kimberly Holden, AuD[a],
Margaret McRedmond, AuD[b]

KEYWORDS

- Pediatric audiology test battery • Cross-check principle • Pediatric case studies

KEY POINTS

- A comprehensive test battery that includes objective tests such as otoacoustic emissions and acoustic reflexes, as well as word recognition, is essential for the diagnosis of hearing disorders in children.
- The cross-check principle relies on both behavioral and physiologic tests to ensure accurate diagnosis of hearing disorders, including retrocochlear pathology.
- A comprehensive audiologic test battery approach is essential to the management of pediatric hearing and language disorders.
- Clinical history and behaviors observed during audiologic evaluation are critical to accurate diagnosis and management of children.

INTRODUCTION

Pediatric audiology is best described as both a science and an art. Science is the foundation of the pediatric hearing evaluation, as outlined in The Joint Committee on Infant Hearing Year 2019 Position Statement.[1] This document summarizes best practice standards for the diagnosis of pediatric hearing loss through literature reviews and expert opinions. However, in the pediatric setting, the process of obtaining behavioral hearing thresholds is as variable as the personalities of the children tested. That is where the *art* of pediatric audiology comes into play. The marriage of science and art in pediatric audiology is embodied in the cross-check principle.

[a] Ann and Robert H. Lurie Children's Hospital of Chicago, 225 East Chicago Avenue, Box 148, Chicago, IL 60611-2605, USA; [b] Vanderbilt University Medical Center, 1215 21st Avenue South Suite 9302, Nashville, TN 37232, USA
* Corresponding author.
E-mail address: jringger@luriechildrens.org

Otolaryngol Clin N Am 54 (2021) 1143–1154
https://doi.org/10.1016/j.otc.2021.08.009
0030-6665/21/© 2021 Elsevier Inc. All rights reserved.

The cross-check principle, first introduced by Jerger and Hayes[2] more than 40 years ago, acknowledges the limitations of a behavioral hearing test in isolation, particularly in the pediatric population. Jerger and Hayes[2] recommended that behavioral results, considered the gold standard, should be "cross-checked" or confirmed by additional test measures. That is, the test battery approach supplements behavioral data that might be inconclusive with information that might be confirmatory or lead to a different diagnosis.

In the decades since Jerger and Hayes[2] first introduced the cross-check principle, technology has expanded the pediatric clinical test battery. **Table 1** outlines the physiologic and behavioral measures now available. Each provides unique and valuable information about the auditory system. The following cases highlight the importance of performing a comprehensive test battery.

CASE 1
History

Abi, a 14-year-old girl, was referred to an otolaryngologist because she reported not hearing well for several months. Her medical and otologic history was otherwise unremarkable. She reported relying on lip reading to understand conversations and was struggling at school. A hearing test showed a mild to moderately severe sensorineural hearing loss (SNHL) with excellent word recognition (>90%) in both ears (**Fig. 1**). Hearing aids, a computed tomographic temporal bone study, and genetic testing were recommended.

At scheduled audiologic testing 6 weeks after the hearing aid fitting, Abi reported little benefit. A repeat hearing test (see **Fig. 1**) revealed bilateral moderately severe to severe SNHL. Her hearing aids were exchanged for more powerful devices. She was referred to an otologist regarding cochlear implant candidacy. As part of that evaluation, a more comprehensive hearing assessment (**Fig. 2**) was performed that included physiologic testing.

Test Battery Results

- Otoscopic evaluation: Unremarkable for both ears
- Tympanometry: Bilateral hypermobility of the tympanic membranes
- Acoustic reflexes: Present at sporadic frequencies (ipsilateral)
- Distortion product otoacoustic emissions (DPOAEs): Present and robust across the frequency range in both ears
- Pure tone audiometry: Profound hearing loss from 250 to 8000 Hz, bilaterally (could not obtain bone conduction due to inconsistent responses)
- Speech reception threshold (SRT): 95 dB HL for both ears
- Word recognition score (WRS):
  - Right ear: 100% when presented at 110 dB HL
  - Left ear: 100% when presented at 110 dB HL

An auditory brainstem response (ABR) was recommended because of poor agreement between objective and behavioral measures and other inconsistencies. ABR results were consistent with normal hearing in both ears.

Discussion

In this case, physiologic test measures were crucial for uncovering inconsistencies and ruling out a hearing loss. Had a comprehensive test battery been performed at the first audiology visit, unnecessary referrals for imaging and genetic testing and purchase of hearing aids would have been avoided.

Table 1
Pediatric audiology test battery

Behavioral Measures	Pure tone audiometry	VRA	Measures hearing thresholds to frequency-specific stimuli. Confirms the type and degree of hearing loss. Test technique will vary based on the patient's age and developmental level
		CPA	
		Conventional audiometry	
	Speech audiometry	SAT/SRT	Measures a hearing threshold for speech. Used to cross-check frequency-specific hearing thresholds
		Speech perception testing	Assesses various levels of auditory perceptual abilities, including pattern perception, discrimination, word recognition, and comprehension
Physiologic measures	Acoustic immittance	Tympanometry	Measures ear canal volume, middle ear admittance, and middle ear pressure using a single-probe frequency
		Acoustic reflexes	Evaluates the integrity of the auditory pathway to the level of the brainstem. Abnormal reflex patterns can help differentiate retrocochlear from cochlear and conductive hearing losses
		Wideband reflectance	Assesses middle ear function across a wide range of frequencies
	Otoacoustic emissions	TEOAEs, DPOAEs	Assesses outer hair cell function in the cochlea. Used in the diagnosis of AN/AS and sensorineural hearing loss
	Evoked potentials	ABR, ASSR, CAEP	Measures a neural response to sound to evaluate auditory system function and estimate hearing thresholds. ABR testing is used in the diagnosis of AN/AS and brainstem auditory pathway dysfunction

Abbreviations: ABR, auditory brainstem response; AN/AS, auditory neuropathy/auditory synaptopathy; ASSR, auditory steady state response; CAEP, cortical auditory evoked potentials; CPA, conditioned play audiometry; DEOAE, distortion product otoacoustic emissions; SAT/SRT, speech awareness/reception threshold; TEOAE, transient evoked otoacoustic emissions; VRA, visual reinforcement audiometry.

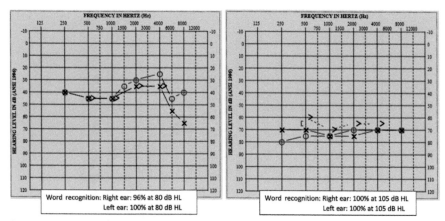

Word recognition: Right ear: 96% at 80 dB HL
Left ear: 100% at 80 dB HL

Word recognition: Right ear: 100% at 105 dB HL
Left ear: 100% at 105 dB HL

Fig. 1. Case 1: First and second hearing test 6 weeks later (left to right).

The following "red flags" were identified by the test battery approach:

- DPOAEs and acoustic reflexes were present in both ears. These findings would have been absent if the patient truly had the degree of SNHL demonstrated by the patient (**Table 2**).
- WRSs were normal bilaterally when they should have been very poor given the profound degree of SNHL demonstrated by the patient.
- Supporting observations by the audiologist:
  - The child did not consistently respond as if she had difficulty hearing during the test procedures. For example, when the audiologist asked, using a normal conversational level, if the acoustic reflex stimuli were too loud, the child immediately answered without requiring repetition or visual cues.

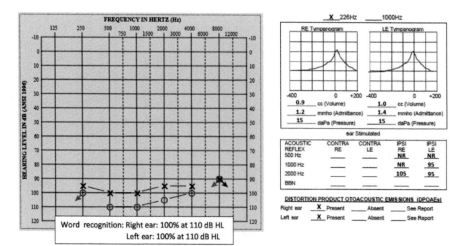

Word recognition: Right ear: 100% at 110 dB HL
Left ear: 100% at 110 dB HL

Fig. 2. Case 1: Comprehensive audiologic evaluation including pure tone audiogram, tympanometry, ipsilateral acoustic reflexes, and otoacoustic emissions.

Table 2	
Acoustic reflex patterns and typical associations with hearing status[4]	
Hearing Status	**Expected Acoustic Reflex Pattern**
Normal hearing (0–25 dB HL)	Present between 75 and 95 dB HL
Cochlear hearing loss	Present at < 60 dB HL sensation level[a] or absent with greater degrees of hearing loss
Retrocochlear pathology	Present at > 100 dB HL sensation level[a] or absent

[a] Decibel level greater than hearing threshold.
Data from Gefand SA, Schwander T, Silman S. Acoustic reflex thresholds in normal and cochlear-impaired ears: effects of no-response rates on 90th percentiles in a large sample. J Speech and Hear Disord 1990;55:198–205.

CASE 2
History

Roberto, a 6-year-old boy, was seen for a hearing aid consultation. His medical history was unremarkable. He had passed newborn hearing screening. More recently, he failed his first 2 school hearing screenings in his left ear. A hearing test at an outside facility included only tympanometry and pure tone audiometry. Results indicated normal hearing in the right ear and a moderate SNHL in the left ear with normal tympanograms, bilaterally. His father reported having long-standing concerns about his son's hearing. He explained that Roberto frequently required repetition and asked for a higher volume on the television. In addition, Roberto's teacher had expressed concern about inattention and disruptive behavior in the classroom. The father was anxious to proceed with amplification for these reasons.

Test Battery Results

A comprehensive audiologic evaluation was performed to confirm the results of Roberto's outside hearing test:

- Otoscopy: Nonoccluding cerumen, bilaterally
- Tympanometry: Normal middle ear mobility in both ears
- Acoustic reflexes: Present in the right ear and absent in the left ear (ipsilateral and contralateral)
- DPOAEs: Robust across the frequency range in both ears
- Pure tone audiometry: Normal hearing sensitivity in the right ear and a moderate SNHL in the left ear, consistent with prior hearing test.
- SRT: 10 dB HL in the right ear and 75 dB HL in the left ear
- WRS:
  - Right ear: 96% at 50 dB HL (40 dB more than the SRT)
  - Left ear: 16% at 95 dB HL (most comfortable level)

Owing to the unexpected finding of DPOAEs in the left ear, and WRSs poorer than expected, there was concern about the possibility of left cochlear nerve deficiency. Hearing aid fitting was deferred, and the child was referred to otolaryngology. MRI confirmed left cochlear nerve deficiency. Amplification of the left ear was not recommended. Classroom accommodations and a future trial with a CROS aid were discussed with the family.

Discussion

The use of a comprehensive test battery approach, including DPOAEs and word recognition testing, revealed important findings not provided by prior testing that included only tympanometry and pure tone audiometry. Cochlear nerve deficiency is one of the most common causes of unilateral hearing loss in childhood, especially for losses in the severe to profound range.[3] DPOAEs might also be present in some children with nerve deficiency. Therefore, these children can pass newborn hearing screening when conducted using technology that relies on otoacoustic emissions. In addition, a subset of patients with this condition present with thresholds in the mild to moderate range associated with poorer discrimination than expected for the degree of hearing loss. For this child, the use of a comprehensive test battery significantly changed the diagnosis and management.

The following "red flags" pointed to a site of lesion distal to the cochlea:

- Although DPOAEs can be present with a mild hearing loss, robust DPOAEs in an ear with moderate SNHL are not expected. This finding points to a site of lesion distal to the inner ear, most likely the cochlear nerve.
- Very poor speech understanding in an ear with only a moderate SNHL is not expected. This finding is also consistent with cochlear nerve deficiency.
- Other relevant observations and teaching points:
  ○ Babies born with cochlear nerve deficiency may have DPOAEs and may, therefore, pass newborn hearing screening using otoacoustic emission technology. Such babies are not expected to pass newborn hearing screening in the affected ears when ABR technology is used.
  ○ With cochlear hearing loss, acoustic reflexes are typically present at a reduced sensation level when thresholds are less than or equal to 50 dB HL (see **Table 2**). The absence of reflexes in this case is expected given the underlying cochlear nerve deficiency. Acoustic reflexes are absent in auditory neuropathy/auditory synaptopathy (AN/AS) and cochlear nerve deficiency, even when auditory thresholds are in the normal to moderate range. It is also important to remember that acoustic reflexes (1) cannot be measured in the presence of conductive hearing loss and (2) are not measurable in ears with pressure equalization (PE) tubes.[5]

CASE 3
History

Casey is an 11-year-old child with a chief complaint of "muffled hearing" and intermittent tinnitus in the right ear, beginning 3 months prior. Her history was negative for acute illness or trauma in the past 6 months. She had passed her newborn hearing screening and previous school hearing screenings. Her otolaryngologist noted a normal examination and referred Casey for audiologic evaluation.

Test Battery Results

A comprehensive evaluation was performed:

- Otoscopic evaluation: Unremarkable for both ears
- Tympanometry: Normal middle ear function, bilaterally
- Acoustic reflexes: Present in the left ear and absent in the right ear (ipsilateral and contralateral)
- DPOAEs: Robust across the frequency range in both ears
- Pure tone audiometry: *Normal hearing in both ears*
- SRT: 10 dB HL in both ears, consistent with pure tone thresholds
- WRS:

- Right ear: 80% at moderate-intensity level (50 dB HL) and 40% at a high-intensity level (80 dB HL)
- Left ear: 96% at moderate-intensity level (50 dB HL) and 100% at a high-intensity level (80 dB HL)

Based on concern for retrocochlear involvement, an MRI was ordered by the otolaryngologist. Results revealed astrocytoma in the posterior fossa causing secondary obstructive hydrocephalus, prompting an urgent referral to neurosurgery.

Discussion

The use of a comprehensive test battery approach provided critical information revealing retrocochlear pathology in an ear that had not yet developed measurable hearing loss. Had only tympanometry and pure tone audiometry been done, this child's tumor diagnosis would have been delayed.

The "red flags" pointing to pathologic condition distal to the cochlea:

- Absence of right ipsilateral and contralateral acoustic reflexes in the context of normal hearing. This finding provides objective data about a problem with integrity of the neural auditory pathway (see **Table 2**).
- Asymmetry of WRSs between the right and left ear. The scores in the right ear are lower than expected. In addition, a decrease in word recognition performance when testing was repeated at a higher intensity level, known as "roll over effect," was observed. This phenomenon is associated with retrocochlear pathology.[6]

Other teaching points:

- Tumors of the eighth nerve or brain causing hearing difficulties are rare during childhood. However, unilateral symptoms, especially in the older child with no history of prior hearing difficulties, is concerning and requires further evaluation. The combination of a thorough history and comprehensive audiologic test battery can identify which children would benefit from imaging.

CASE 4
History

Jack, a 7-year-old boy, was referred to audiology by his primary care physician for hearing concerns. His past medical history was unremarkable. His parents reported observing the following: (1) they often need to repeat themselves when communicating with their son, (2) he often mishears or misunderstands statements, and (3) he becomes upset when more than one person speaks at the same time while he is listening to conversation. In addition, his parents reported that Jack's first-grade teacher had concerns about his hearing in class. Jack was struggling to learn to spell and to read. He had already repeated prekindergarten due to concerns regarding academic readiness. Jack was receiving speech therapy in school to address an articulation disorder and was making little progress.

Test Battery Results

A comprehensive audiologic evaluation was performed (**Fig. 3**):

- Otoscopic evaluation: Unremarkable for both ears
- Tympanometry: Normal for both ears
- Acoustic reflexes: Absent ipsilateral acoustic reflexes for both ears
- DPOAEs:
  - Right ear: Present and robust

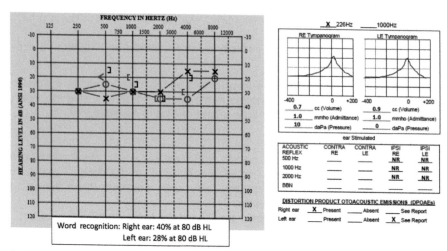

Fig. 3. Case 4 demonstrating a mild sensorineural hearing loss for the right ear and a mild mixed hearing loss for the left ear.

- o Left ear: Present from 2000 to 3000 Hz and reduced or absent from 4000 to 8000 Hz
- Pure tone audiometry: Mild bilateral hearing loss rising to normal hearing in the high frequencies; sensorineural in the right ear and mixed in the left ear
- SRT: Consistent with the pure tone audiometry bilaterally
- WRS:
  - o Right ear: 40% when presented at 80 dB HL
  - o Left ear: 28% when presented at 80 dB HL

Absent ipsilateral reflexes, present DPOAEs, and poor word recognition bilaterally in the presence of only a mild SNHL suggest the possibility that Jack could have AN/AS (Linda J. Hood and article, "Auditory Neuropathy / Auditory Synaptopathy," in this issue). He was referred for an unsedated ABR, which confirmed AN/AS, bilaterally (Fig. 4). An MRI of the brain, cochleae, and eighth nerves was normal. He was referred for cochlear implant evaluation.

Discussion

About 7% to 10% of children with SNHL have AN/AS.[7] AN/AS significantly impacts speech perception, especially when background noise is present. This special population may not benefit, or receive less than expected benefit, from amplification. Therefore, counseling and management of AN/AS often requires a different approach than typical SNHL. These children often benefit from cochlear implantation.

The following are the "red flags" that raised suspicion for AN/AS:

- Acoustic reflexes should be present with mild to moderate SNHL (see **Table 2**). The absent reflexes without another explanation (conductive pathology or PE tubes that would interfere with reflex measurement) is concerning for AN/AS.[8]
- The presence of robust DPOAEs in ears with mild SNHL is unusual. Although DPOAEs can be present with mild SNHL, it is rare, and the robust responses in the right ear would not be expected.[9]
- WRSs were significantly poorer than expected with mild hearing loss. Children with a mild hearing loss usually have good to excellent word understanding and, therefore, typically do well with amplification.

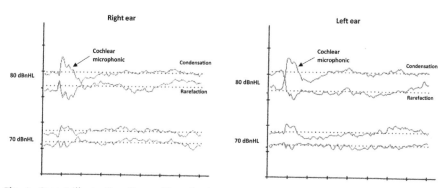

Fig. 4. Case 4 illustrating the auditory brainstem response with cochlear microphonics present bilaterally.

- Other observations of significance and teaching points:
  - The degree of hearing difficulty described by the parent is disproportionate to the degree of hearing loss; this may be a sign of AN/AS.
  - Over time, DPOAEs can disappear in some children with AN/AS; this may be more likely for those fitted with amplification.[10]
  - Children with AN/AS and middle ear disease can be more difficult to identify because DPOAEs generally cannot be measured when middle ear effusion is present. The presence of PE tubes can also interfere with the accurate recording of DPOAEs.

CASE 5
History

Paul is a 28-month-old boy with speech delay referred to audiology to rule out hearing loss before a speech and language evaluation. His mother has no concerns about his hearing. She reports that he is "in his own little world" but does respond to things that interest him. Paul says a few words including "mama" and "dada and, occasionally, understands instructions given without a gesture. He passed an ABR hearing screening at birth.

Test Battery Results
- Otoscopic evaluation: Unremarkable for both ears
- Tympanometry: Normal middle ear mobility in both ears
- Acoustic reflexes: Could not obtain due to patient behavior
- DPOAEs: Present responses across the frequency range. A tablet playing songs was used to distract child during testing
- Visual reinforcement audiometry (VRA): Minimum response levels in the normal hearing range at 2000 Hz and in the mild hearing loss range at 500 Hz in the soundfield (not ear specific)
- Speech awareness threshold: Normal hearing range in the soundfield

The audiologist noted the following behaviors: poor eye contact, toe walking, atypical vocalizations, fixation on his hands, and distress when his ears were touched. Based on these observed behaviors, the audiologist administered the Modified Checklist for Autism in Toddlers, Revised (M-CHAT-R)[11] and asked his mother the following questions:

- How does he play? *Answer:* Lines up cars; likes to spin and watch wheels
- Are there things he does that are unusual or odd? *Answer:* Fascinated with light switches and will turn them on or off for an hour if allowed
- Does he throw a lot of temper tantrums? *Answer:* About 3 per day; becomes upset when something happens outside of his routine
- Does he have sensitivity issues with food, clothes, or sounds? *Answer:* Only eats 3 different foods, has trouble keeping clothes on, dislikes hair and teeth brushed
- How does he communicate that he wants something? *Answer:* Pushes parent to what he wants and puts the parent's hand on it.

Paul received a score of 7 on the M-CHAT, placing him at medium risk for autism spectrum disorder (ASD). These results were reviewed with the mother and a comprehensive autism evaluation was recommended. She was counseled that audiologic results, although limited, indicated that hearing was likely not the reason for his speech delay. An ABR confirmed normal hearing bilaterally. Further evaluations confirmed the ASD diagnosis.

Discussion

Delayed speech and language are often the first concerns evaluated when children have atypical development. Because a hearing test is generally recommended before a child's initial speech and language evaluation, audiologists often see children with ASD and other disorders of development before they receive a formal developmental evaluation. In addition to using a comprehensive audiologic test battery, the history and clinical observations obtained by the audiologist in this case led to expansion of the evaluation process because of concerns about ASD. Use of measures such as the M-CHAT in combination with physiologic test measures that are part of a comprehensive audiologic battery might obviate ABR evaluation.

The "red flags" during this evaluation were not the result of discrepancies in test results that comprise the test battery. Rather the "red flags" were a constellation of behaviors recognized by the pediatric audiologist as concerning for ASD in light of the child's age and speech delay:

- During VRA threshold testing, child responded to speech stimuli in the normal hearing range but was far less interested in frequency-specific stimuli.
- Headphones or insert phones in the ear canal could not be used to obtain ear-specific information because the child became distressed when his ears were touched.
- Child demonstrated poor eye contact, toe walking, and atypical vocalizations.
- Other teaching points:
  ○ ASD might be the cause of speech and language delay of young children referred for audiologic evaluation. Experienced pediatric audiologists can recognize behaviors concerning for ASD diagnosis.
  ○ Individual ear testing might be challenging in children with ASD. ABR might be necessary for confirmation of normal hearing bilaterally.

SUMMARY

As medical professionals, it is important to provide quality care to all, but especially to pediatric patients unable to describe their symptoms. A comprehensive audiologic test battery approach distinguishes unexpected test results from routine findings, which may uncover an underlying diagnosis and optimize management. This approach is especially important when applied to evaluations of infants and young children who require early intervention to enhance development of language and cognition.

The cases presented herein highlight the importance of a thorough audiologic evaluation. In each case, if only pure tone audiometry and tympanometry were done, each child would have been misdiagnosed or a disorder would have gone undetected. Word recognition testing helped to identify a brain tumor, auditory neuropathy, and a malingerer. Acoustic reflexes and DPOAEs were influential in differentiating cochlear from retrocochlear pathology. In the case of the brain tumor, a detailed case history prompted the audiologist to test for roll over with word recognition testing. The audiologist's observations of behavior were also important in providing a recommendation for an autism evaluation.

Pediatric audiology relies on carefully selected, evidence-based test measures and the art of obtaining test results from young patients who are not forthcoming with their audiometric information. The importance of the cross-check principle outlined decades ago still holds true today.

CLINICS CARE POINTS

- Appropriate use of a comprehensive audiologic test battery, including physiologic measures, can help to identify:
  - Auditory neuropathy/auditory synaptopathy
  - Feigning of hearing loss
  - Eighth nerve pathology such as nerve deficiency and tumors
  - Sensorineural versus conductive hearing loss
  - Presence of a hearing loss versus developmental delay
- Pediatric audiologists' scope of practice includes screening for developmental concerns. Behavioral hearing testing gives the audiologist the opportunity to identify atypical behaviors and screen for developmental disorders.
- The diagnosis of AN/AS should be considered in children with communication disorders, especially those with a diagnosis of SNHL and unexpectedly poor speech perception despite fitting of amplification.
- Unilateral AN/AS can be associated with cochlear nerve deficiency, especially if auditory thresholds are in the severe to profound range. Noncontrast imaging by MRI that includes high-resolution imaging of the internal auditory canals can confirm this diagnosis.

DISCLOSURE

The authors have no commercial or financial conflicts of interest or any funding sources in relation to the article.

REFERENCES

1. The J Committee on Infant Hearing. Year 2019 position statement: principles and guidelines for early hearing detection and intervention programs. J Early Hearing Detect Intervention 2019;4(2):1–44.
2. Jerger JF, Hayes D. The cross-check principle in pediatric audiometry. Arch Otolaryngol 1976;102(10):614–20.
3. Clemmens CS, Guidi J, Caroff A, et al. Unilateral cochlear nerve deficiency in children. Otolaryngol Head Neck Surg 2013;149(2):318–25.

4. Gefand SA, Schwander T, Silman S. Acoustic reflex thresholds in normal and cochlear-impaired ears: effects of no-response rates on 90th percentiles in a large sample. J Speech Hear Disord 1990;55:198–205.
5. Northern JE, Gabbard SA. Acoustic reflex. In: Katz JA, editor. Handbook of clinical audiology. 4th edition. LW&W; 1994. p. 302–3.
6. Jerger J, Jerger S. Diagnostic significance of PB word functions. Arch Otolaryngol 1971;93(6):573–80.
7. Roush PA. Children with auditory neuropathy spectrum disorder. In: Seewald ER, Tharpe AM, editors. Comprehensive handbook of pediatric audiology. San Diego: Plural Publishing; 2011. p. 734–50.
8. Kitao KY, Mutai H, Namba Ka, et al. Deterioration in distortion product otoacoustic emission in auditory neuropathy patients with distinct clinical and genetic backgrounds. Ear Hear 2019;40(1):184–91.
9. Smith Joanna T, Wolfe Jace. Testing otoacoustic emissions in children: the known, and the unknown. Hearing J 2013;66(12). https://doi.org/10.1097/01.HJ. 0000441062.09162.be.
10. Berlin1 Charles I, Hood Linda J, Morlet Thierry, et al. Absent or elevated middle ear muscle reflexes in the presence of normal otoacoustic emissions: a universal finding in 136 cases of auditory neuropathy/dys-synchrony. J Am Acad Audiol 2005;16(8):546–53.
11. Yuen T, Penner M, Carter MT, et al. Assessing the accuracy of the Modified Checklist for Autism in Toddlers: a systematic review and meta-analysis. Dev Med Child Neurol 2018;60(11):1093–100.

Overview of Medical Evaluation of Unilateral and Bilateral Hearing Loss in Children

Sampat Sindhar, MD, MSCI, Judith E.C. Lieu, MD, MSPH*

KEYWORDS

- Hearing loss • Children • Etiology • Diagnostic test • Diagnostic imaging

KEY POINTS

- Detection of hearing loss in children occurs at multiple points of care, although newborn hearing screening is the most universal.
- Obtaining a history and performing a physical examination, after obtaining an audiogram, are the first steps in the evaluation of any child with hearing loss.
- Evaluation of hearing loss is variable, depending on age, acuity of presentation, and other concomitant patient factors.
- Treatment of the underlying etiology, when possible, may halt or improve hearing loss, and infectious etiology should be identified early.

INTRODUCTION/HISTORY/DEFINITIONS/BACKGROUND

Epidemiology

Pediatric hearing loss (HL) is a common childhood disability. Approximately 1.1/1000 to 1.7/1000 newborns have permanent bilateral severe to profound HL, and another 1/1000 to 2/1000 newborns have mild to moderate bilateral or unilateral HL.[1,2] By the age of 19 years, 15% to 18% of children may develop HL due to delayed-onset HL, trauma, ototoxic medication exposures, and infection.[3] Among children with HL, 95% have normal hearing parents, making counseling and education vital to the management of the child with HL.[4]

HL classifications are broad and are included in **Box 1**. Among children with HL, sensorineural HL (SNHL) accounts for 68% of bilateral HL and 45% of unilateral HL; conductive HL (CHL) accounts for only 7% of bilateral HL and 30% of unilateral HL.[2]

Unlike HL in adults, childhood HL often occurs before speech and language develop, adversely affecting a child's academic success and quality of life.[5,6] Thus, the main impetus for early identification and treatment of HL has been to prevent speech-language delay and subsequent consequences.

Department of Otolaryngology-Head and Neck Surgery, Washington University School of Medicine in St. Louis, 660 South Euclid Avenue, Campus Box 8115, St. Louis, MO 63110, USA
* Corresponding author.
E-mail address: lieujudithe@wustl.edu

Otolaryngol Clin N Am 54 (2021) 1155–1169
https://doi.org/10.1016/j.otc.2021.07.005
0030-6665/21/© 2021 Elsevier Inc. All rights reserved.

Box 1
Classification of hearing loss

SNHL: HL that results from dysfunction in transmitting the neural signal within the cochlea, cochlear nerve, brainstem, and/or auditory cortex, or dysfunction along the pathways that connect those structures

CHL: HL that results from dysfunction in transmitting the acoustic signal to the cochlea, usually within the external or middle ear, including the external auditory canal, tympanic membrane, middle ear cavity, and ossicles

Mixed HL: HL that combines aspects of SNHL and CHL

ANSD: also referred to as auditory neuropathy spectrum disorder or auditory dys-synchrony, it is diagnosed when cochlear function is present but sounds are not transmitted normally to the brain. It is considered a subtype of SNHL. Otoacoustic emissions derived from the cochlea typically are present but auditory brainstem responses are absent with preservation of the cochlear microphonic.

Severity of HL
  Slight—hearing thresholds 16–25 dB
  Mild—hearing thresholds 26–40 dB
  Moderate—hearing thresholds 41–55 dB
  Moderately severe—hearing thresholds 56–70 dB
  Severe—hearing thresholds 71–90 dB
  Profound—hearing thresholds >90 dB

Currently, diagnostic medical evaluation of HL varies significantly. A recent cross-sectional study of children with any degree of SNHL found that only approximately 27% received any diagnostic testing for the evaluation of HL, and 25% received any medical intervention in the form of speech-language pathology referral, hearing aid evaluation, or cochlear implantation. Significant disparities in diagnostic testing depended on whether the evaluation was performed by a pediatrician or general practitioner, general otolaryngologist, or pediatric otolaryngologist. Pediatric otolaryngologists were the most likely to order genetic testing for patients.[7] This review focuses on the medical evaluation of HL with a proposed algorithm.

Newborn Hearing Screening

Newborn hearing screening (NHS) began as targeted screening of neonatal intensive care unit graduates and infants with known risk factors for HL, to achieve early identification and habilitation of children with congenital HL.[8] The passage of the Newborn and Infant Hearing Screening and Intervention Act of 1999 facilitated universal NHS in all 50 states. The average age of HL detection decreased from 2.5 years to 14 months as a result.[9] The advent of universal NHS using otoacoustic emissions and automated auditory brainstem response, combined with early intervention services (Individuals with Disabilities Education Act, 2004, Part C), educational assistance through individualized educational plans for those with HL (Individuals with Disabilities Education Act, 2004, Part B), and hearing technologies, including cochlear implantation and digital hearing aids, have allowed a majority of children with HL to enroll in inclusionary school environments and maximize their speech-language skills.

Identification of Hearing Loss in Early Childhood and Adolescence

Although universal NHS has led to earlier identification and management of HL, children with later-onset HL often are missed. Among children with SNHL due to congenital cytomegalovirus (CMV), half are identified through NHS whereas the remainder experience delayed-onset of HL.[10] Subsequent to passing NHS, there are several points of care at which a child with later-onset HL might come to medical attention: preschool and school hearing screenings, pediatrician well-child visits, and parent-initiated evaluation for concerns about hearing and/or speech-language development.

Aside from UNHS, HL detection in childhood and adolescence is highly variable. Parental suspicion for HL tends to underestimate HL, with the notable exceptions of unilateral HL and HL that is consistent across frequencies (ie, flat audiogram), at which parents may be surprisingly adept at identifying[11] prior to their child's physician.[12] In general, postnatally acquired HL often initially is suspected through hearing screening done at school or by the primary care physician during well child care. In the United States, however, only 34 states require school-based hearing screening, whereas the remaining 17 states recommend school-based screening. Only 20 of 34 states require screening beyond the sixth grade, to capture HL in the junior high or high school years.[13] School-based hearing screening involves pure tone audiometry testing at 1000 Hz, 2000 Hz, and 4000 Hz at 20 dB or 25 dB.[14] Only 2 states (Kansas and Colorado) require 6000-Hz testing for children in the fourth grade or above.[13]

Failing a school screening does not mean that hearing is evaluated. A study evaluating failure rate and referral patterns in multiple pediatrician practices incorporating greater than 1000 patients found that despite 10% of children failing hearing screening at well-child visits, more than half (59%) of children did not have their hearing rechecked and were not referred for further evaluation.[15] Although children who fail hearing screening could have normal hearing or temporary loss that resolves, physicians should maintain a high degree of suspicion for permanent HL and ensure audiologic testing is completed, especially if a parent expresses concerns about hearing difficulties, speech or language delay, or worsened academic performance.

Purpose of Medical Evaluation

The medical evaluation of HL is conducted for many reasons. Parents and family members frequently ask why a child has HL. For many children with CHL and some children with SNHL, hearing can be restored fully or partially if the cause can be identified and treated. Occasionally, HL may be the first observed manifestation of an underlying systemic or genetic disease; recognition of the underlying condition can lead to treatment that extends beyond intervening for HL.

Identification of a suspected etiology is possible in 50% to 60% of cases.[16] Depending on the etiology, a patient or family can be counseled on the likelihood of progressive or bilateral HL, such as with congenital CMV infection or enlarged vestibular aqueduct (EVA) syndrome. Information about associated features is another advantage of an etiologic evaluation, for example, Usher syndrome, which is associated with blindness from retinitis pigmentosa. Knowledge of this diagnosis provides an opportunity for evaluation and counseling by ophthalmologic specialists and for parents to keep abreast of research on developing medical treatments. Additionally, identification of an underlying gene mutation can guide reproductive counseling for the patient and family members.

Because evaluation of HL has different purposes and impacts, the timing of testing may vary. When ascertainment of etiology is crucial to intervene or preserve function, testing should be prioritized. For example, a definitive diagnosis of congenital CMV made within the first 3 weeks of life enables the option of antiviral treatment to preserve hearing. Due to the ubiquitous nature of endemic CMV, a diagnosis made after 3 week of age is considered likely due to community exposures and thus postnatal. An infant with bilateral profound SNHL should have an electrocardiogram (ECG) to rule out Jervell and Lange-Nielsen syndrome, an uncommon disorder that can result in

---

Box 2

Etiologies of conductive hearing loss visible on computed tomography

Neoplasm: facial nerve paraganglioma or hemangioma

Persistent stapedial artery

Missing oval window

Congenital stapes ankylosis

Malleus bar (associated with congenital aural atresia)

---

sudden death due to long QT syndrome. Alternatively, when ascertainment of etiology does not alter the recommended intervention, testing can be deferred. To exemplify, genetic testing for an infant with bilateral profound SNHL and no suspicion for syndromic HL may be deferred until after initial hearing aid fitting, early intervention, and/or cochlear implantation has been initiated.

INITIAL EVALUATION
Evaluation of Conductive Hearing Loss

CHL typically occurs when sound transmission to the inner ear through the ear canal and middle ear is impeded. Children with CHL have similar clinical presentation in terms of parental concerns and developmental impact as children with SNHL and may have variable onset during childhood. Although estimates of CHL prevalence are difficult to ascertain, acute otitis media (AOM) and otitis media with effusion (OME) are the most common causes of childhood HL. AOM and OME causes temporary and fluctuating CHL with more limited long-term impact on language development.[17] The management of persistent OME associated with CHL has been discussed broadly in the otolaryngology community[18] and this review focuses on permanent CHL.

Evaluation of permanent CHL requires a thorough history and a detailed physical examination of the ear (**Table 1**). Examination of the outer ear should include identification of ear pits, tags, and malformations of the pinna. The ear canal and middle ear space should be assessed for external ear canal stenosis, cerumen impaction, debris, or foreign body. The tympanic membrane should be assessed for perforation, effusion, or cholesteatoma.

Minor malformations of the middle ear also may lead to HL. To define surgical anatomy and determine surgical candidacy, most investigators recommend temporal bone high-resolution computed tomographic (CT) imaging.[19] Although problems in the external ear often are visible on otoscopic examination, imaging may aid in confirming the diagnosis and defining extent of disease. Temporal bone CTs are essential to diagnosis of cholesteatoma not visible on otoscopic examination and may provide evidence of congenital ossicular malformations or otosclerosis.[20–22] CT imaging of ears with congenital ossicular fixation may be normal, however, due to joint fixation. Third window phenomenon causing pure CHL is uncommon but may be seen in superior and posterior semicircular canal dehiscence and X-linked stapes gusher syndrome (DFNX2), which is associated with dilated internal auditory canal. A conductive component (mixed HL) attributed to the third window effect is not uncommon in ears with EVA.[23–25] In addition, children with cochlear malformation are more likely to develop SNHL after head trauma. Therefore, when evaluating children with congenital CHL or sudden HL due to head trauma, cochlear malformation should be

Table 1	
Initial medical evaluation: historical risk factors and physical examination findings	
Patient History Risk Factors	**Physical Examination Findings**
Perinatal history: TORCH (toxoplasmosis, other (syphilis), rubella, cytomegalovirus, and herpes simplex) infections, hypoxic injury, prematurity, low birthweight, hyperbilirubinemia, exposure to ototoxic medications Medical history: bacterial meningitis, head trauma, noise exposure, exposure to ototoxic medications (eg, history of malignancies), seizures, choanal atresia Comorbid conditions: congenital heart disease, sickle cell disease, renal disease, ophthalmologic abnormalities, known chromosomal abnormalities, Family history: first-degree and second-degree relatives with childhood-onset or adolescent-onset HL Developmental history: social and language development, motor milestone development	Hypernasal speech External ear: microtia, aural atresia, pits or tags, cerumen impaction, mass, foreign body, external auditory canal cholesteatoma Middle ear: tympanic membrane perforation, tympanic membrane retraction (eg, incudostapediopexy, adhesion to the promontory), middle ear fluid (any type), middle ear mass or cholesteatoma Facial features: upsloping or down-sloping palpebral fissures, flattened malar eminences, hypertelorism, white forelock (patchy depigmentation of hair/skin) Eyes: heterochromic irides, coloboma Oral cavity: cleft lip and/or cleft palate, submucous cleft palate Neck: cysts, pits, or tags Cardiac: murmurs Vestibular function: standing on 1 foot with eyes open and eyes closed variations, tandem standing, head thrust, dynamic visual acuity

suspected. Similarly, stapes abnormalities, such as congenital stapes footplate fixation, and otosclerosis, are rare but should be suspected in the setting of family history of CHL and prior stapedectomy. Identification of temporal bone abnormalities on CT can improve the planning and counseling for surgical interventions, such as ossicular reconstructions or extirpation of cholesteatoma.

Up to 30% of children with congenital ear deformities have an inherited syndrome. Among the more common are branchio-oto-renal syndrome, Treacher Collins syndrome, and Klippel-Feil syndrome.[26] Branchio-oto-renal syndrome, also known as Melnick-Fraser syndrome, also can present with SNHL or mixed HL. Physical examination findings of preauricular pits, defects in the external or middle ear, and branchial cleft anomalies are highly suggestive of this syndrome, and kidney abnormalities on renal ultrasound can confirm the diagnosis. Treacher Collins syndrome, also known as mandibulofacial dysostosis, includes physical findings of down-slanting palpebral fissures, malar and mandibular hypoplasia, microtia, and CHL.[27] Four gene loci produce the phenotypic expression of this syndrome, with dominant inheritance and variable penetrance. Klippel-Feil syndrome is associated with several gene loci with autosomal dominant or recessive inheritance and can be associated with CHL, SNHL, or mixed HL; microtia; and cleft palate. Fused cervical vertebrae produce the appearance of short neck and limited neck range of motion.

For children with CHL, nonurgent CT imaging should be obtained after appropriate rehabilitation has begun, as discussed later. Children with features suggestive of a syndromic CHL should undergo genetic counseling or testing to uncover other associated medical issues that could affect a child's health and development.

Evaluation of Sudden Sensorineural Hearing Loss

Evaluation for sudden HL is a special circumstance where urgent evaluation and treatment may differentiate between a reversible or permanent HL. History and physical examination are key to guiding which diagnostic tests should be considered and performed. Because sudden HL is rare in children, adult guidelines based on predominantly autoimmune mediated HL often are followed.[28] Autoimmune HL is less common in children, however, compared with other etiologies. More common etiologic categories include infection and congenital inner ear malformations. For example, both unilateral and bilateral sudden HL may be caused by Lyme disease, mumps, Epstein-Barr virus, herpes simplex virus (HSV) (Ramsay Hunt syndrome), syphilis, and delayed-onset congenital CMV infection. Diagnostic testing at time of onset of HL is available for all but delayed-onset congenital CMV. Identification of an infectious etiology may enable medical treatment to stabilize hearing. For children with delayed-onset HL due to congenital CMV, antiviral therapy is not effective. A diagnosis may be obtained, however, by requesting testing of their neonatal dried blood spot (DBS), also known as a Guthrie card. The DBS is collected for neonatal screening, which does not include congenital CMV. The DBS is stored by state health departments for variable periods of time and may be available for CMV testing. Diagnosis of congenital CMV also may be supported by findings of characteristic intracranial abnormalities on CT or MR imaging. Unrecognized inner ear malformations, of which EVA is the most common, may be the cause of sudden SNHL. Temporal bone CTs identify EVA, whereas MR imaging reveals enlargement of the endolymphatic duct and sac. Effectiveness of steroid therapy, either orally or intratympanic application, for sudden loss due to EVA is unproved.

Evaluation of Sensorineural or Mixed Hearing Loss

Whereas CHL often is due to an underlying anatomic etiology, SNHL has multiple etiologies, including infectious, anatomic, genetic, traumatic, ototoxic, and autoimmune. The prevalence of these underlying causes changes depending on the age of presentation of HL.

In general, infectious causes of HL have decreased due to widespread vaccination globally. The incidence of congenital rubella has decreased due to vaccinations, and CMV, and toxoplasmosis also have decreased over time even without a vaccine; however, congenital syphilis has resurged in some communities.[29] Acquired SNHL can occur with measles, mumps, varicella zoster, Lyme disease, Zika, bacterial meningitis, and, rarely, otitis media. Lyme disease and toxoplasmosis are endemic in some regions and nonexistent in other regions. Travel exposures can help distinguish risk for Zika, measles, and Lyme disease, among others. Childhood vaccination history may illuminate those who are at risk for mumps, measles, and bacterial meningitis due to Streptococcus pneumonia.

Genetic evaluation for SNHL has become complicated with the constantly increasing number of genes and pathogenic mutations. **Table 2** shows a partial list of nonsyndromic and syndromic HL genetic loci. Nonsyndromic HL generally is bilateral and often autosomal recessive. According to the Hereditary Hearing Loss Homepage, 123 nonsyndromic HL genes have been identified as 2/5/2021.[30] The genetic work-up and current commercially available testing has been published in the literature[31] and is discussed in Genetics of Childhood Hearing Loss by Cynthia Casson Morton and Calli Ober Mitchell.

Children with syndromic HL may not have obvious additional physical findings and, therefore, may not be identified at initial evaluation by an otolaryngologist. Alternatively, children with syndromic HL may be identified by other medical subspecialists

Table 2
Some common nonsyndromic and syndromic genetic hearing loss genes[37]

Nonsyndromic Genetic Cause/Locus	Associated Genes	Common Findings	Additional Diagnostic Findings
DFNB1 (OMIM 220290)	GJB2 GJB6	Congenital mild to profound autosomal recessive nonsyndromic HL	Usually, normal temporal bone imaging.[38] Rarer dominant forms are associated with skin disease. Uncommon digenic inheritance with both GJB2 and GJB6
DFNB16 (OMIM 603720)	STRC (CATSPER2)	Bilateral mild to moderate congenital SNHL. Deletion of both STRC and CATSPER2 is associated with SNHL and male infertility	
DFNA8/12 (OMIM 602574)	TECTA	Often prelingual, and often milder and mid-frequency or high-frequency SNHL	
DFNB21 (OMIM 602574)	TECTA	Prelingual severe to profound SNHL	
DFNB3 (OMIM 600316)	MYO15 A	Progressive bilateral SNHL	
Mitochondrial HL (OMIM 561000)	MT-RNR1; 1555G > A (this is the most common one)	Maternally inherited nonsyndromic HL or HL that occurs after brief exposure to aminoglycosides	There also are many mitochondrial syndromes, some of which include HL
Syndromic HL			
Pendred syndrome (recessive) (OMIM 274600)	SLC26A4	Euthyroid (often) goiter, progressive, often asymmetric, mild to moderate SNHL or mixed HL	Intracochlear partition defect type II (Mondini) deformity, in which the cochlea has less than the normal 2.5 turns, and/or EVA on CT or MR imaging

(continued on next page)

Table 2
(continued)

Nonsyndromic Genetic Cause/Locus	Associated Genes	Common Findings	Additional Diagnostic Findings
Usher syndrome (recessive) (OMIM 276900, 276904, 601067, 602083, 606943) (OMIM 276901, 605472, 611383) (OMIM 276902)	MYO7A USH1C CDH23 PCDH15 SANS/USH1G USH2A ADGRV1 WHRN CLRN1	Type I: profound HL at birth, vestibular dysfunction starting at birth, vision problems early in life Type II: moderate to severe HL at birth, vision problems by adolescence with progression, normal balance Type III: progressive HL, later-onset vestibular dysfunction, and vision loss starting later in childhood or adolescence	Electroretinogram or dark, adapted thresholds may show signs of retinitis pigmentosa earlier than routine ocular examination. There are also few mutations that result in either nonsyndromic RP or nonsyndromic HL.
Alport syndrome (X-linked, recessive, dominant) (OMIM 301050, 203780, 104200)	COL4A5 COL4A3 COL4A4	Progressive HL, hematuria, ocular abnormalities (anterior lenticonus, retinopathy)	Kidney biopsy may reveal glomerulonephritis
Jervell and Lange-Nielsen syndrome (recessive) (OMIM 220400, 612347)	KCNQ1 KCNE1	Severe to profound bilateral congenital HL, syncope, sudden death	Prolongation of QT interval on ECG
Waardenburg syndrome (dominant or recessive) (OMIM 606597, 193510, 602229, 608890, 277580, 613265)	PAX3-WS1/3 MITF – WS2 SNAI2- WS2D SOX10-WS2E, 4C EDNRB- WS4A EDN3-WS$B	HL generally congenital, may be unilateral or bilateral, and can be associated with structural inner ear anomalies, such as EVA. Waardenburg syndrome type 3, and Waardenburg syndrome types 4A and 4B can be autosomal dominant or recessive.	Dystopia canthorum (Waardenburg syndrome type 1), synophrys, vitiligo, heterochromia iridis, white forelock. Upper limb anomalies (Waardenburg syndrome type 3), Hirschsprung disease (Waardenburg syndrome type 4)
Branchio-oto-renal syndrome (dominant) (OMIM 601653, 601205, 600963)	EYA1, SIX1, SIX5	HL generally is congenital; ear anomalies may involve external, middle, and inner ear.	Renal anomalies may be structural, functional, or both

Abbreviation: OMIM, Online Mendelian Inheritance in Man database; CT, computed tomography; EVA, enlarged vestibular aqueduct; HL, hearing loss; MRI, magnetic resonance imaging; SNHL, sensorineural hearing loss.

Permission to reprint from "Hearing Loss in Children: A Review" JAMA. 2020;324(21):2195 to 2205. doi:10.1001/jama.2020.17647 obtained from AMA.

due other anatomic features or abnormalities. Pendred syndrome is the most common syndrome associated with HL, which is secondary to EVA and cochlear malformations. The associated HL is progressive and may be asymmetric. Euthyroid or hypothyroid goiter may occur with Pendred syndrome and could require monitoring of thyroid function. Genetic testing confirms the diagnosis with mutations in the SLC26A4 gene. The perchlorate discharge test, done prior to availability of genetic diagnosis, no longer is used.

Usher syndrome has a multitude of genetic loci with several phenotypes based on the onset/progression of HL and vision loss. When Usher syndrome is suspected due to family history, genetic testing as well as ophthalmologic examination, ideally by a retinal specialist, should be obtained. As noted previously, for children with bilateral profound SNHL, an ECG to rule out Jervell and Lange-Nielsen syndrome, an autosomal recessive disorder defined by accompanying long QT syndrome that can lead to sudden death, is valuable at initial evaluation. Children suspected of having Alport syndrome may have microscopic hematuria on urinalysis before a renal biopsy confirms glomerulonephritis. Although molecular genetic testing is preferred, skin and kidney biopsy also can make the diagnosis of Alport syndrome.

Waardenburg syndrome is among the most heterogeneous of genetic syndromes, with highly variable type, onset, and severity of HL, as well as many different genetic loci. Patchy depigmentation of the hair and skin can be observed, as well as heterochromia irides.

Various forms of trauma are associated with acquired SNHL or mixed HL in children. Temporal bone fractures can result in SNHL due to direct involvement of the cochlear or vestibular apparatus or to concussive head injury without fracture. Barotrauma can occur from any rapid change in pressures in the external ear canal that are not matched in the middle ear due to eustachian tube dysfunction, such as with flying, scuba-diving, or from blast injuries. Diagnosis is based on history of associated activities or exposures.

Increased concern for noise-induced HL among children has been expressed frequently, particularly with the widespread use of headphones and earbuds associated with personal music equipment. Diagnosis is suggested by the finding of progressive high-frequency SNHL often accompanied by tinnitus. Evaluation for these forms of trauma resulting in HL usually requires CT and/or MR imaging to rule in or rule out an abnormality that suggests a different etiology.

As a result of increasingly sophisticated and aggressive medical treatment of life-threatening diseases, ototoxic exposures from therapeutic medications leading to HL have become more frequent. Well known are the associations with aminoglycoside antibiotics, for which some children may have genetic susceptibility due to mitochondrial mutations (see **Table 2**). The use of loop diuretics, such as furosemide; salicylates; antibiotics, such as vancomycin and the macrolides; and antimalarial agents (quinine, chloroquine, and hydroxychloroquine), also have been shown to be associated with HL. Among childhood survivors of malignancies, antineoplastic agents, especially cisplatin and other platinum-based agents, are well-known to be causes of SNHL. It is possible that some children with these exposures may have other temporal bone anomalies that predispose them to HL, so temporal bone imaging via CT or MR imaging is a reasonable diagnostic test to consider. Mechanisms of Ototoxicity & Otoprotection by Peter S. Steyger.

Environmental exposures to heavy metals, including arsenic, cadmium, lead, and mercury, have been found to be associated with higher risk of HL in adolescents. Cadmium and lead, presumed to be associated with electronic-waste pollution, also have been associated with higher prevalence of HL in preschool children in China.[32,33] In children with developmental delays in addition to HL and possible environmental exposures due to where their homes and schools are located, testing of blood levels for these heavy metals may be warranted.

Finally, SNHL can occur as a result of a variety of autoimmune and inflammatory diseases in children (**Table 3**). Although rare, diagnosis can lead to effective treatment and preservation of hearing. Consultation with rheumatology is highly recommended.

Evaluation of Auditory Neuropathy Spectrum Disorder

Auditory neuropathy spectrum disorder (ANSD) often accompanied by a history of hyperbilirubinemia, perinatal hypoxia, prematurity, and low birthweight. ANSD also

Table 3
Autoimmune disease or vasculitides associated with hearing loss[39-46]

Name	Other Affected Systems	Tests
Cogan syndrome (AD)	Eye (interstitial keratitis) Aortitis Systemic	Clinical diagnosis
Kawasaki disease (V)	Mucocutaneous Cardiac (coronary arteritis) Skin (rash) Lymphadenopathy Systemic	Diagnostic criteria
Granulomatosis with polyangiitis (former Wegener granulomatosis (V)	Upper respiratory tract Pulmonary Cardiac Renal Systemic	ANCAs Biopsy
EGPA, formerly Churg-Strauss syndrome (V)	Nasal polyposis Chronic OME Asthma	ACR diagnostic criteria
Systemic lupus erythematosus (AD)	Any organ system, commonly Skin, joints, kidneys Systemic	ANAs, sdDNA, ENAs
Inflammatory bowel disease (Crohn, ulcerative colitis) (AD)	Gastrointestinal inflammation Growth failure Systemic	Clinical features, imaging, endoscopy
Juvenile idiopathic arthritis (AD)	Fever Rash Arthritis	Diagnosis of exclusion
Vogt-Koyanagi-Harada disease (AD)	Eye (uveitis) Skin (vitiligo, alopecia, poliosis) Central nervous system (meningeal signs, cerebrospinal fluid pleocystosis) Systemic	Revised diagnostic criteria proposed by the International Nomenclature Committee

Abbreviations: ACR, American College of Rheumatology; AD, autoimmune disease; ANA, antinuclear antibody; ANCA, antineutrophil cytoplasmic antibody; sdDNA, double-stranded DNA antibody; EGPA, eosinophilic granulomatosis with polyangiitis; ENA, extractable nuclear antigens; V, vasculitides.

may occur on a genetic basis. The most frequent causes of nonsyndromic ANSD are mutation of the OTOF, DFNB59, and DIAPH3 genes. Audiological findings consistent with ANSD also may be seen in children with cochlear nerve aplasia or hypoplasia, often referred to as cochlear nerve deficiency. Evaluation for cochlear nerve deficiency requires high-resolution 3-dimensional MR imaging of the internal auditory canals, because CT temporal bone anatomy may be normal.

DISCUSSION

This overview focuses on etiologic evaluation of children with a definitive diagnosis of HL. Several other algorithms for diagnostic evaluation have been proposed, taking into account diagnostic efficiency and cost considerations.[34–36] Once HL has been confirmed, targeted evaluation for most etiologies of HL is guided by history and physical examination. Diagnostic testing is urgent when the HL is of sudden onset or progresses rapidly, guided by whether suspected etiologies are treatable or involve other organ systems. In general, CT or MR imaging is the most likely diagnostic test to identify an abnormality that either explains the HL or affects the interventions to be recommended. For parents of children with bilateral severe to profound SNHL, next-generation genetic testing is most likely to provide useful information.

SUMMARY
Clinics Care Points

- Evaluation as soon as an infant is identified with HL (**Fig. 1**)
  - Rule out congenital infections that can be treated medically.
  - For children with bilateral profound SNHL, obtain ECG to rule out Jervell and Lange-Neilsen syndrome.
  - For children with suspected syndromic HL, obtain genetic evaluation or consult.

- Evaluation that can be deferred in nonprogressive HL detected in infancy (see **Fig. 1**)
  - Imaging of temporal bone
  - Genetic testing
  - Ophthalmologic examination

- Evaluation for permanent CHL (**Fig. 2**)
  - If sudden onset or progression, obtain urgent CT and consider exploratory tympanotomy.
  - Otherwise, obtain CT/MR imaging at a convenient time
  - Genetic consultation if family history for HL is present
  - Ophthalmologic examination

- Evaluation for sudden SNHL (**Fig. 3**)
  - HSV culture of ear lesions to rule out Ramsay-Hunt, mumps, measles, Lyme disease titer, syphilis
  - CT/MR imaging to rule out cochlear malformation
  - Laboratory evaluation for autoimmune disease or other systemic disease, based on symptoms and physical findings

- Evaluation for bilateral or unilateral SNHL (see **Fig. 3**)
  - CT/MR imaging (MR imaging preferred when goal is to rule out nerve deficiency in unilateral HL)
  - Genetic testing (bilateral or unilateral with suspected syndrome) or consultation
  - DBS evaluation for congenital CMV
  - Ophthalmologic examination

- Further management of all patients
  - Referral to appropriate specialist depending on diagnostic test findings or suspicion of syndromic HL

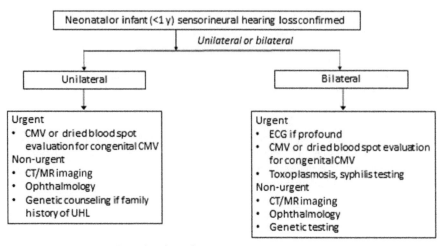

Fig. 1. Diagnostic test algorithm for infant HL.

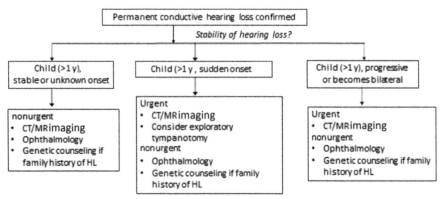

Fig. 2. Algorithm for evaluating permanent CHL.

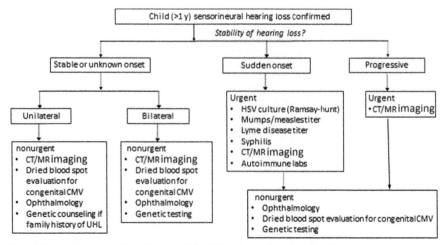

Fig. 3. Diagnostic test algorithm for child SNHL, including sudden SNHL.

DISCLOSURES

JECL is coinventor of the HEAR-QL, a series of hearing-related quality-of-life surveys for children, and receives royalties for their licensed use, which are managed by the Office of Technology Management at Washington University School of Medicine.

REFERENCES

1. Butcher E, Dezateux C , Cortina-Borja M, Knowles RL. Prevalence of permanent childhood hearing loss detected at the universal newborn hearing screen: Systematic review and meta-analysis. PLoS One 2019;14(7):e0219600.
2. 2017 CDC EDHI Hearing Screening & Follow-up Survey (HFHS). 2017 Summary of Diagnostics Among Infants Not Passing Hearing Screening Web site. 2019. Available at: https://www.cdc.gov/ncbddd/hearingloss/2017-data/documents/2017-HSFS_Type-and-Severity-Table.pdf. Accessed July 9, 2021.
3. Wang J, Sung V, Carew P, et al. Prevalence of childhood hearing loss and secular trends: a systematic review and meta-analysis. Acad Pediatr 2019;19(5):504–14.
4. Mitchell RE, Karchmer MA. Chasing the mythical ten percent: parental hearing status of deaf and hard of hearing students in the United States. Sign Lang Stud 2004;4(2):138–63.
5. Lieu JEC. Permanent unilateral hearing loss (UHL) and childhood development. Curr Otorhinolaryngol Rep 2018;6(1):74–81.
6. Vila PM, Lieu JE. Asymmetric and unilateral hearing loss in children. Cell Tissue Res 2015;361(1):271–8.
7. Qian ZJ, Chang KW, Ahmad IN, Tribble MS, Cheng AG. Use of diagnostic testing and intervention for sensorineural hearing loss in US children from 2008 to 2018. JAMA Otolaryngol Head Neck Surg 2021;147(3):253–60.
8. Joint Committee on Infant Hearing 1994 Position Statement. American Academy of Pediatrics Joint Committee on infant hearing. Pediatrics 1995;95(1):152–6.
9. Harrison M, Roush J, Wallace J. Trends in age of identification and intervention in infants with hearing loss. Ear Hear 2003;24(1):89–95.
10. Fowler KB, Dahle AJ, Boppana SB, Pass RF. Newborn hearing screening: will children with hearing loss caused by congenital cytomegalovirus infection be missed? J Pediatr 1999;135(1):60–4.
11. Watkin PM, Baldwin M, Laoide S. Parental suspicion and identification of hearing impairment. Arch Dis Child 1990;65(8):846–50.
12. Harrison M, Roush J. Age of suspicion, identification, and intervention for infants and young children with hearing loss: a national study. Ear Hear 1996;17(1):55–62.
13. Sekhar DL, Zalewski TR, Paul IM. Variability of state school-based hearing screening protocols in the United States. J Commun Health 2013;38(3):569–74.
14. Harlor AD, Bower C. Medicine CoP, Ambulatory, Surgery SoO-H, Neck. Hearing assessment in infants and children: recommendations beyond neonatal screening. Pediatrics 2009;124(4):1252–63.
15. Halloran DR, Wall TC, Evans HH, Hardin JM, Woolley AL. Hearing screening at well-child visits. Arch Pediatr Adolesc Med 2005;159(10):949–55.
16. Cushing SL, Papsin BC. Taking the History and Performing the Physical Examination in a Child with Hearing Loss. Otolaryngol Clin North Am 2015;48(6):903–12.
17. Gravel JS, Wallace IF. Effects of otitis media with effusion on hearing in the first 3 years of life. J Speech Lang Hear Res 2000;43(3):631–44.

18. Rosenfeld RM, Shin JJ, Schwartz SR, et al. Clinical practice guideline: Otitis media with effusion (update). Otolaryngol Head Neck Surg 2016;154(1 Suppl): S1–41.
19. Dougherty W, Kesser BW. Management of conductive hearing loss in children. Otolaryngol Clin North Am 2015;48(6):955–74.
20. Curtin HD. Imaging of conductive hearing loss with a normal tympanic membrane. AJR Am J Roentgenol 2016;206(1):49–56.
21. DeMarcantonio M, Choo DI. Radiographic evaluation of children with hearing loss. Otolaryngol Clin North Am 2015;48(6):913–32.
22. Lipschitz N, Kohlberg GD, Scott M, Greinwald JH. Imaging findings in pediatric single-sided deafness and asymmetric hearing loss. Laryngoscope 2020; 130(4):1007–10.
23. Arjmand EM, Webber A. Audiometric findings in children with a large vestibular aqueduct. Arch Otolaryngol Head Neck Surg 2004;130(10):1169–74.
24. Govaerts PJ, Casselman J, Daemers K, De Ceulaer G, Somers T, Offeciers FE. Audiological findings in large vestibular aqueduct syndrome. Int J Pediatr Otorhinolaryngol 1999;51(3):157–64.
25. Nakashima T, Ueda H, Furuhashi A, et al. Air-bone gap and resonant frequency in large vestibular aqueduct syndrome. Am J Otol 2000;21(5):671–4.
26. Bartel-Friedrich S, Wulke C. Classification and diagnosis of ear malformations. GMS Curr Top Otorhinolaryngol Head Neck Surg 2007;6:Doc05.
27. Online Mendelian Inheritance in Man. In: National Center for Biotechnology Information, U.S. National Library of Medicine. 2020. Available at: https://www.ncbi. nlm.nih.gov/omim. Accessed July 9, 2021.
28. Chandrasekhar SS, Tsai Do BS, Schwartz SR, et al. Clinical Practice Guideline: Sudden Hearing Loss (Update). Otolaryngol Head Neck Surg 2019; 161(1_suppl):S1–45.
29. Cuffe KM, Kang JDY, Dorji T, et al. Identification of US Counties at Elevated Risk for Congenital Syphilis Using Predictive Modeling and a Risk Scoring System. Sex Transm Dis 2020;47(5):290–5.
30. Van Camp GSR. Hereditary Hearing Loss Homepage. 2020. Available at: https:// hereditaryhearingloss.org. [Accessed 3 June 2020].
31. Belcher R, Virgin F, Duis J, Wootten C. Genetic and Non-genetic Workup for Pediatric Congenital Hearing Loss. Front Pediatr 2021;9:536730.
32. Shargorodsky J, Curhan SG, Henderson E, Eavey R, Curhan GC. Heavy metals exposure and hearing loss in US adolescents. Arch Otolaryngol Head Neck Surg 2011;137(12):1183–9.
33. Liu Y, Huo X, Xu L, et al. Hearing loss in children with e-waste lead and cadmium exposure. Sci Total Environ 2018;624:621–7.
34. Preciado DA, Lawson L, Madden C, et al. Improved diagnostic effectiveness with a sequential diagnostic paradigm in idiopathic pediatric sensorineural hearing loss. Otol Neurotol 2005;26(4):610–5.
35. Preciado DA, Lim LH, Cohen AP, et al. A diagnostic paradigm for childhood idiopathic sensorineural hearing loss. Otolaryngol Head Neck Surg 2004;131(6): 804–9.
36. Liming BJ, Carter J, Cheng A, et al. International Pediatric Otolaryngology Group (IPOG) consensus recommendations: Hearing loss in the pediatric patient. Int J Pediatr Otorhinolaryngol 2016;90:251–8.
37. Lieu JEC, Kenna M, Anne S, Davidson L. Hearing Loss in Children: A Review. JAMA 2020;324(21):2195–205.

38. Kenna MA, Rehm HL, Frangulov A, Feldman HA, Robson CD. Temporal bone abnormalities in children with GJB2 mutations. Laryngoscope 2011;121(3):630–5.
39. Espinoza GM, Wheeler J, Temprano KK, Keller AP. Cogan's Syndrome: Clinical Presentations and Update on Treatment. Curr Allergy Asthma Rep 2020;20(9):46.
40. Magalhães CM, Magalhães Alves NR, Oliveira KM, Silva IM, Gandolfi L, Pratesi R. Sensorineural hearing loss: an underdiagnosed complication of Kawasaki disease. J Clin Rheumatol 2010;16(7):322–5.
41. Bohm M, Gonzalez Fernandez MI, Ozen S, et al. Clinical features of childhood granulomatosis with polyangiitis (wegener's granulomatosis). Pediatr Rheumatol Online J 2014;12:18.
42. Seccia V, Fortunato S, Cristofani-Mencacci L, et al. Focus on audiologic impairment in eosinophilic granulomatosis with polyangiitis. Laryngoscope. 2016; 126(12):2792–7.
43. Paraschou V, Chaitidis N, Papadopoulou Z, Theocharis P, Siolos P, Festas C. Association of systemic lupus erythematosus with hearing loss: a systemic review and meta-analysis. Rheumatol Int 2021;41(4):681–9.
44. Wengrower D, Koslowsky B, Peleg U, et al. Hearing Loss in Patients with Inflammatory Bowel Disease. Dig Dis Sci 2016;61(7):2027–32.
45. El-Gharib AM, El-Barbary AM, Aboelhawa MA, Elkholy RM. Audiovestibular function in patients with juvenile idiopathic arthritis (JIA). Acta Otolaryngol 2016; 136(10):1058–63.
46. Lavezzo MM, Sakata VM, Morita C, et al. Vogt-Koyanagi-Harada disease: review of a rare autoimmune disease targeting antigens of melanocytes. Orphanet J Rare Dis 2016;11:29.

Comprehensive Audiological Management of Hearing Loss in Children, Including Mild and Unilateral Hearing Loss

Kathryn Wiseman, PhD[a], Caitlin Sapp, PhD[b],
Elizabeth Walker, PhD[b], Ryan McCreery, PhD[a],*

KEYWORDS

- Children with hearing loss • Amplification candidacy • Device selection
- Hearing aid verification • Outcome validation

KEY POINTS

- Timely diagnosis of childhood hearing loss should include prompt referrals (eg, medical, language) and recommendations for audiological intervention based on type, degree, and configuration of hearing loss.
- If a child is a candidate for amplification, the audiologist should work with the family to select a hearing technology, with consideration of device style, advanced features, and compatibility with assistive technology.
- Ongoing verification of amplification ensures that speech sounds amplified by the hearing aid are audible but not too loud, especially as a child grows and ear canal acoustics change.
- Audiologists should validate hearing aids using parental questionnaires and aided speech perception measures to assess the benefit of amplification for auditory and speech-language development.

Once hearing loss (HL) is confirmed, referrals for medical and language intervention should be made immediately. A full medical workup by a pediatric otolaryngologist is indicated anytime HL is diagnosed. This evaluation helps rule out transient conductive issues, ensures that a child's ears are healthy enough for hearing aids, and could reveal related conditions. The findings of a medical examination complement audiometric findings and may influence the technology recommendations. Specific recommendations for audiological intervention will depend on the type, degree, and

[a] Boys Town National Research Hospital, 555 N 30th Street, Omaha, NE 68131, USA; [b] University of North Carolina Medical Center, 435 Meadowmont Village Circle, Chapel Hill, NC 27517, USA
* Corresponding author. Wendell Johnson Speech and Hearing Center, 250 Hawkins Drive, Iowa City, IA 52242.
E-mail address: Ryan.McCreery@boystown.org

Otolaryngol Clin N Am 54 (2021) 1171–1179
https://doi.org/10.1016/j.otc.2021.08.006
0030-6665/21/© 2021 Elsevier Inc. All rights reserved.

oto.theclinics.com

configuration of HL. If an HL is permanent or unlikely to be resolved through medical management, amplification should be considered as part of the intervention whether the loss is sensorineural, conductive, or mixed. Any degree of HL can negatively impact spoken language development,[1,2] so amplification should be considered if a child has thresholds that are more than the normal levels for any frequencies that are important for understanding speech. Unilateral HL can impact access to binaural cues that are important for localization of sound and listening in noise, so children with mild to severe unilateral HL should also be considered candidates for amplification. Conventional audiometric testing in dB HL (decible hearing level) can produce threshold values that are enhanced by a child's small ear canal size, particularly for insert earphones.[3] In cases in which infants or children with small ear canals present with mild degrees of HL, audiologists may convert the dB HL audiogram to dB sound pressure level (SPL) to evaluate the effects of threshold elevation on speech audibility and weigh the potential audibility benefits of providing hearing aids.[4] Children with severe or profound degrees of HL might receive limited benefit from amplification and eventually be evaluated for cochlear implant candidacy.[5] However, hearing aids provided before cochlear implantation have demonstrated benefits for postimplantation outcomes,[6] so auditory stimulation via hearing aids is often recommended for children with severe to profound degrees of HL, even when the potential for long-term benefits are low.

SELECTION OF HEARING DEVICES

Once a child is determined to be a candidate for amplification, the audiologist and family work together to select hearing technology that is audiologically appropriate and flexible enough to accommodate a child's changing needs over time. Several clinical and nonclinical factors will influence what hearing aid they select.

STYLE

The most common style of hearing aid for infants and children is a behind-the-ear (BTE) hearing aid, coupled with an earmold. Different sizes of BTE models provide the audiologist with a wide range of power options to produce appropriate amplification for HL ranging from mild to severe. BTE devices can be reprogrammed to accommodate some progression in hearing sensitivity. When the pinna is substantial enough to support the weight and size of a BTE hearing aid, it should be considered the first choice for infants and children. As a child's ear grows, the earmold can be remade to ensure an adequate fit without having to replace the device. For older children and teens with normal low-frequency hearing, the audiologist and family might choose to pursue an open-fit BTE or receiver-in-the-ear device to reduce occlusion.

EARMOLDS

An earmold is a custom-fitted mold of the pinna and ear canal that connects with the BTE hearing aid via soft tubing and delivers amplified sound to the ear. Earmolds require that a set of ear impressions be taken and mailed (or scanned and sent) to an earmold fabrication laboratory. The audiologist makes these impressions by mixing and placing fast-setting material into the canal and concha. This process can take place under sedation if a child undergoes a sedated auditory brainstem response (ABR) to establish their level of HL. Earmolds come in several materials, and families are able to choose from a wide range of colors and designs. Soft earmold materials, such as silicone, are currently the standard of care for pediatric patients, because they ensure a comfortable fit in a wide variety of environments and can be easily modified. Harder earmold materials like acrylic and vinyl are longer lasting than soft materials and can be a good option in cases of allergy to silicone.

Without a tightly fitting earmold, sound can leak out of the ear canal and reenter the device's microphones. This leakage creates acoustic feedback audible as a whistling sound to those in close proximity to a child with hearing aids. Excessive feedback should be addressed, because it indicates poor acoustic coupling that can lead to insufficient amplification. In the first year of life, a family can expect several visits to remake and fit new earmolds. If a child's ear has grown such that an earmold needs to be replaced, the audiologist should remeasure the child's ear canal acoustics using the real-ear-to-coupler-difference (RECD) procedure.

TECHNOLOGY LEVELS

Hearing aid manufacturers often market devices at several technological levels (at progressively higher cost), ranging from introductory devices to premium technology devices. Although the connotation of higher cost is often higher performance, research on premium hearing technology does not bear this out. The additional cost of premium-level technology is often not justified based on available research in children. **Table 1** contains a summary of available technology and the most recent evidence-based recommendations for their use.[7]

COMPATIBILITY

Children with HL often rely on assistive technology such as remote-microphone systems to supplement their amplification in acoustically adverse environments like classrooms. Families and audiologists must think ahead about features a child might need during the lifespan of their device (typically 3–5 years). For example, some hearing aids might not be compatible with the remote-microphone systems used in school settings. Although school districts are required to find solutions in such cases, careful selection at the time of fitting can prevent long periods of poor auditory access in the classroom due to incompatibility.

HEARING AID FUNDING

A final important factor in selecting a hearing device for a young child is funding. At the time of this writing, 17 US states have passed legislation that makes pediatric hearing aid insurance coverage mandatory; however, even in states with coverage mandates, there are exceptions. Other states have no such mandate and families can face steep out-of-pocket costs that can be a barrier to timely amplification.[8] State Medicaid programs cover amplification for children whose families meet qualification standards but place a heavy administrative burden on accessing these benefits or have limited funding. Families must use a provider who has enrolled in their state's Medicaid program and agreed to accept Medicaid rates for amplification services, which may force some providers not to provide care due to poor reimbursement rates. To fill gaps in pediatric hearing aid funding, hearing professionals can compile a reference of charitable and alternative funding mechanisms available within their state.

VERIFICATION

Once the appropriate device is selected, the hearing aid must be programmed and fit to the individual child. The fitting processes include teaching the child and their family

Table 1
Advanced hearing aid features and their recommendation status in current pediatric amplification guidelines[7]

Advanced Feature	Description	Considerations for Pediatric Use
Directional microphones	Digital processing strategies based on positional cues relative to hearing aid microphones meant to emphasize the amplification of sounds from the front	Careful consideration should be taken before activating directional microphones because of the importance of listening through overhearing or incidental learning for children. Automatic directionality is preferable to manual directionality
Feedback suppression	Algorithms that detect acoustic feedback and limit gain for high frequencies to resolve it	Feedback suppression should be activated in pediatric devices
Amplitude compression	Varies amplification based on the loudness of the incoming signal. Compression promotes the use of a listener's full range of hearing	Compression improves audibility for soft speech and maintains comfort for loud inputs

Data from American Academy of Audiology (2013). Clinical practice guidelines: Pediatric amplification. Reston, VA.

about daily use and care of the devices, as well as hearing aid verification. The goal of hearing aid verification is to ensure that speech sounds amplified by a hearing aid are audible, but not too loud, using objective acoustic measurements. If speech sounds are not audible, children who are learning spoken language might be at risk for receiving inadequate audibility and experiencing poorer language outcomes.[4,9] Audiologists must assess hearing aid fit relative to pediatric prescriptive targets and determine the audibility of speech at the initial fitting appointment and at regular intervals as the child grows (less than 1 year old: every 3 months; less than 3 years old: every 6 months; older than 3 years: every year). Verification should also be performed after any changes to a child's hearing thresholds, hearing aids, or earmolds. Verifying hearing aids helps ensure that speech remains audible as the child grows and ear canal acoustics change.

Audiologists perform hearing aid verification using a probe microphone system. This system evaluates sound levels produced by a hearing aid in response to various levels of speech input by measuring hearing aid output (**Fig. 1**). In children who can sit for multiple measurements, hearing aid output is measured directly in the ear canal using a small flexible probe tube microphone placed near the eardrum just beyond the hearing aid. Alternatively, clinicians can record the child's RECD, which is a quick measurement of a child's ear canal acoustics, and use those values across multiple measures to verify hearing aid output within a hearing aid test box. Age-related average values can also be used if a child's RECDs cannot be measured; however, average RECDs lack the specificity of individually measured values.

Performing probe microphone measurements allows audiologists to assess if hearing aid output meets levels prescribed by pediatric-fitting formulas (eg, desired sensation level) for soft, average, and loud speech inputs (eg, 55–75 dB SPL). These evidence-based formulas suggest optimal hearing aid output levels based on a child's

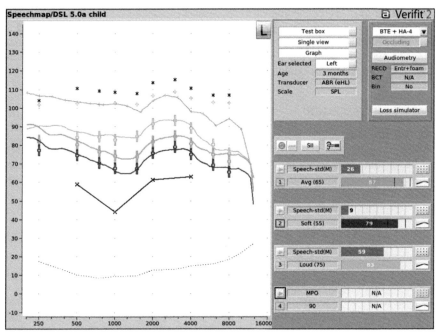

Fig. 1. A sound pressure level (SPL) o-gram for a child with mild to moderate hearing loss. Blue X symbols connected with a blue line represent the audiometric thresholds in dB SPL for the left ear. Crosses represent prescriptive targets for soft (pink), average (green), and loud (teal) input levels for speech. The orange line represents the maximum power output of the hearing aid. The unaided speech intelligibility indices (SIIs) for each input level are shown as gray bars in the legend on the right, and the aided SII for each input level is represented by the corresponding colored bar. The comparison of unaided and aided SIIs shows the change in audibility with amplification for each input level.

age and hearing levels. Fitting output to these targets can help achieve consistent speech audibility.[10] In addition, audiologists should ensure that the maximum power output of the hearing aid is not uncomfortably loud. Furthermore, advanced hearing aid features (see **Table 1**) can be verified using the probe microphone system or the coupler. Verification of these features should occur if these features are activated to avoid negative impact on audibility.

Clinicians also determine aided audibility of speech by looking at the speech intelligibility index (SII).[11] The SII quantifies the proportion of speech that is audible and useable by the listener, ranging from no access (SII = 0) to complete access to speech (SII = 1). The aided SII is calculated by summing the sensation level (ie, difference in hearing aid output levels relative to child's unaided hearing levels) of frequency bands that are weighted by the amount of speech information that each band provides. Although aided audibility is not a direct measure of speech understanding, it reflects the weighted proportion of speech signals that is audible. On average, children with better aided audibility have better language[12] and speech recognition abilities[13] than those with poorer audibility.

Measuring aided audibility helps inform clinicians, parents, and professionals of a child's strengths and challenges related to accessing speech (eg, ability to hear high-frequency phonemes like /s/; access to soft, distant speech). Monitoring is particularly important for children with progressive HL, because hearing aid gain might need to be adjusted more frequently. If a child's SII is low or if the hearing aids fail to meet targets, clinicians should consider changes to a child's intervention that increase audibility, such as hearing aid reprogramming to meet prescriptive targets, fitting more powerful hearing aids, or cochlear implantation.

HEARING AID VALIDATION

In addition to hearing aid verification, progress with amplification needs to be documented through validation. Validation confirms that a child's communication needs are being met. Two types of validation are commonly recommended for children: parental questionnaires and aided speech perception assessment. Both provide important information about how a child is performing with hearing aids.[7]

PARENT QUESTIONNAIRES

Parent-report questionnaires can inform us about children's development in audition and spoken communication, both preintervention and postintervention. These questionnaires cover infancy through adolescence, although they are typically used in the birth to 3-year age range, when children are unable to self-report. Parents can complete questionnaires on their own or via an interview with a clinician. The LittlEARS[14] and the Parents' Evaluation of Aural/Oral Performance of Children (PEACH)[15] are two examples of valid and reliable questionnaires that ask parents to assess their child's functional auditory skills (eg, "Does your child react to his/her name?"). Repeated administration of these questionnaires can help clinicians track auditory skill development over time (see Ref.[16] for a review of parent-report tools).

AIDED SPEECH PERCEPTION ASSESSMENT

Aided speech perception assessment is another important validation tool that tells us how a child uses amplification to support listening and spoken language. Speech awareness can be assessed during infancy. Starting around 18 months, most children can participate in aided detection or discrimination tasks. The Ling Six Sound Test[17] is a commonly used assessment of a child's ability to detect or discriminate specific speech sounds that cover the long-term average speech spectrum. Speech recognition can be assessed with familiar words or sentences. If children are limited in their language production skills, they can be encouraged to point to real objects or pictures. Once a child has achieved ceiling levels on speech recognition in quiet, background noise can be added to the testing scenario. The addition of background noise offers a more ecologically valid approach to speech recognition, compared with listening in quiet.

Poor speech recognition performance can be due to several factors. Language and cognitive abilities can affect speech recognition, so children with cognitive-linguistic delays might have lower scores on a speech perception test than children who have stronger skills in these areas. Auditory access can also impact speech perception performance. If a child is demonstrating very low scores on an aided speech recognition test, and the test has been deemed appropriate for the child's language and cognitive level, the audiologist should use probe microphone measures to verify the audibility provided by the hearing aid. Because children show wide variation in speech perception skills, conducting assessments at each audiology appointment can assist in understanding the development of auditory skills in an individual child.

AIDED SOUND FIELD THRESHOLDS OR FUNCTIONAL GAIN

Another option for validating hearing aid fittings is to measure a listener's audiometric thresholds through a loudspeaker while wearing the hearing aids. This approach, known as aided sound field thresholds or functional gain, can tell us whether amplification leads to improvements in audiometric thresholds compared with an unaided audiogram. Although it might seem intuitive to validate amplification using aided sound field thresholds, there are numerous limitations to this approach that preclude the use of this procedure in contemporary practice. The signal processing in hearing aids affects the perception of the tones we use during an aided audiogram, leading to responses that are not reflective of speech audibility. Furthermore, being able to detect very soft sounds in a sound booth does not fully explain how a child is able to understand conversational level speech in real-life situations. The only time that aided sound field testing is appropriate for validation is for children who use bone conduction devices or cochlear implants. Both forms of hearing technology bypass the typical air conduction route for hearing and, therefore, preclude the measurement of aided speech audibility.

IMPACT OF HEARING AID USE ON LANGUAGE ACQUISITION

A child with typical hearing is expected to show steady growth in language skills over time, making 1 year of language growth over 12 months. Young children with HL can start off with delays compared with children with typical hearing, so they need to show faster language growth (more than 1 year of language growth over 12 months) to close that gap. For families that choose a listening and spoken language approach, hearing aids are a tool for closing that gap. A recent longitudinal study of 317 children with mild to severe HL found that increased hearing aid use had a positive effect on language growth rates. That is, children who wore hearing aids more often throughout the day displayed steeper change in language scores over time, whereas children who wore hearing aids less showed a flat trajectory.[9] More specifically, children who wore hearing aids 10 or more hours a day made more than a year's worth of language gains in a year's time, essentially closing the gap between themselves and children with typical hearing. In contrast, children who wore their hearing aids for less than 10 hours a day showed no change in their rate of language growth (ie, the gap between their language skills compared with average performance for same-aged children with typical hearing remained the same over time). Furthermore, amount of daily hearing aid use predicts language outcomes for children with HL, regardless of the degree of HL. In other words, children with mild HL showed as much benefit from hearing aids as children with severe HL.[18] These results provide strong evidence for the importance of consistent hearing aid use for achieving maximum benefits from auditory stimulation, particularly during important periods of early brain development.

DISCLOSURE

This paper was supported by a grant from NIH R01 DC013591 (PI McCreery).

CLINICS CARE POINTS

- Accurate and timely diagnosis of HL sets the stage for informed management recommendations, including amplification, if appropriate.

- Selection of hearing devices by the audiologist, child, and family should account for the individual child's age, audiological profile, and educational needs.
- Verification and validation of the fitted devices ensure that the child has access to audible speech of a variety of input levels and that the devices are providing benefit via auditory and speech perception outcomes.
- Consistent use of well-fit hearing aids facilitates auditory access, which leads to improved outcomes for children with HL.

REFERENCES

1. Davis JM, Elfenbein J, Schum R, et al. Effects of mild and moderate hearing impairments on language, educational, and psychosocial behavior of children. J Speech Hear Disord 1986;51(1):53–62.
2. Tharpe AM. Unilateral and mild bilateral hearing loss in children: past and current perspectives. Trends Amplif 2008;12(1):7–15.
3. Voss SE, Herrmann BS. How does the sound pressure generated by circumaural, supra-aural, and insert earphones differ for adult and infant ears? Ear Hear 2005 1;26(6):636–50.
4. McCreery RW, Walker EA, Stiles DJ, et al. Audibility-based hearing aid fitting criteria for children with mild bilateral hearing loss. Lang Speech Hear Serv Sch 2020;51(1):55–67.
5. Carlson ML, Sladen DP, Gurgel RK, et al. Survey of the American Neurotology Society on cochlear implantation: part 1, candidacy assessment and expanding indications. Otol Neurotol 2018;39(1):e12–9.
6. Nickerson A, Davidson LS, Uchanski RM. Pre-implant hearing aid fittings and aided audibility for pediatric cochlear implant recipients. J Am Acad Audiol 2019;30(8):703.
7. American Academy of Audiology (2013). Clinical practice guidelines: pediatric amplification. Reston, VA.
8. McManus MA, Levtov R, White KR, et al. Medicaid reimbursement of hearing services for infants and young children. Pediatrics 2010 1;126(Supplement 1): S34–42.
9. Tomblin JB, Harrison M, Ambrose SE, et al. Language outcomes in young children with mild to severe hearing loss. Ear Hear 2015;36(0 1):76S.
10. McCreery RW, Walker EA, Spratford M, et al. Longitudinal predictors of aided speech audibility in infants and children. Ear Hear 2015;36:24S–37S.
11. American National Standards Institute (ANSI).S3.5-1997 R-2007, American National standards methods for the calculation of the speech intelligibility index. New York: American National Standards Institute; 2007.
12. Stiles DJ, Bentler RA, McGregor KK. The speech intelligibility index and the pure-tone average as predictors of lexical ability in children fit with hearing aids. J Speech Lang Hear Res 2012;55(3):764–78.
13. McCreery RW, Walker EA, Spratford M, et al. Speech recognition and parent ratings from auditory development questionnaires in children who are hard of hearing. Ear Hear 2015;36(1):60S–75S.
14. Coninx F, Weichbold V, Tsiakpini L, et al. Validation of the LittlEARS® Auditory Questionnaire in children with normal hearing. Int J Pediatr Otorhinolaryngol 2009;73(12):1761–8.
15. Ching TY, Hill M. The parents' evaluation of aural/oral performance of children (PEACH) scale: normative data. J Am Acad Audiol 2007;18(3):220–35.

16. Bagatto MP, Moodie ST, Seewald RC, et al. A critical review of audiological outcome measures for infants and children. Trends Amplification 2011;15(1): 23–33.
17. Ling D. Speech development in hearing-impaired children. J Commun Disord 1978;11(2–3):119–24.
18. Tomblin JB, Oleson JJ, Ambrose SE, et al. The influence of hearing aids on the speech and language development of children with hearing loss. JAMA Otolaryngol Head Neck Surg 2014;140(5):403–9.

Expansion of Audiologic Criteria for Pediatric Cochlear Implantation

Christine Brown, AuD, René H. Gifford, PhD*

KEYWORDS

- Pediatric audiology • Hearing aids • Cochlear implants • Implant candidacy
- Speech recognition

KEY POINTS

- Children with better than bilateral severe-to-profound sensorineural hearing loss and better than 30% aided word or sentence recognition achieve significant benefit from cochlear implantation.
- On the basis of published data, children with an unaided pure tone average > 60 dB HL should be referred for cochlear implant evaluation.
- Limiting cochlear implant candidacy to children with bilateral profound or severe-to-profound sensorineural hearing loss as outlined in outdated Food and Drug Administration–approved indications is not aligned with current outcomes research and best clinical practice.

INTRODUCTION

Cochlear implants (CIs) have dramatically impacted communication, education, and quality of life for children with severe-to-profound sensorineural hearing loss. Just a few decades ago, children born with profound deafness were routinely sent to a residential school for the deaf to acquire language, socialization, and academic instruction. Today, children with congenital deafness are routinely implanted at 12 months of age or younger and are capable of achieving age-appropriate speech, language, and preliteracy skills before entering a mainstream kindergarten.[1] To this end, CIs have been termed the most successful sensory neuroprostheses of all time.[2,3]

In June 1990, the Food and Drug Administration (FDA) approved CIs for children ≥2 years with bilateral profound sensorineural hearing loss. The minimum age for FDA-labeled CI indications was later lowered to 18 months in 1998, 12 months in 2000, and 9 months in 2020. The latest age adjustment for pediatric CI candidacy

Department of Hearing and Speech Sciences, Vanderbilt University Medical Center, 1215 21st Avenue South, 9302 MCE South Tower, Nashville, TN 37232, USA
* Corresponding author.
E-mail address: rene.gifford@vumc.org

Otolaryngol Clin N Am 54 (2021) 1181–1191
https://doi.org/10.1016/j.otc.2021.08.002
0030-6665/21/© 2021 Elsevier Inc. All rights reserved.

took 2 decades, despite considerable evidence for CI benefits as early as 6 months of age on development of auditory skills, speech, and language.[4-8]

In addition to age, there are audiometric criteria and aided speech recognition criteria for older children capable of completing speech perception tasks. Currently, all FDA-approved systems list bilateral profound sensorineural hearing loss in their labeled indications; however, since 2000, Cochlear Americas Corporation has also listed bilateral severe-to-profound hearing loss for children ≥ 2 years. As of July 2019, there is also an FDA-approved indication for cases of single-sided deafness (SSD) and asymmetric hearing loss for children ≥ 5 years (MED-EL); however, SSD and highly asymmetric hearing losses are beyond the scope of this article.

With respect to aided speech perception, pediatric CI candidates were originally expected to demonstrate no evidence of open-set speech recognition with appropriately fitted hearing aids (HAs). Current labeling at this time specifies 12% to 30% aided word recognition (Advanced Bionics [AB]: <12%; Cochlear <30%; MED-EL: <20%) or up to 30% sentence recognition (AB) for pediatric CI candidacy.[9-11] Paradoxically, pediatric CI criteria are more restrictive than adult indications. Specifically, adults can demonstrate a bilateral moderate sloping-to-profound sensorineural hearing loss with aided sentence recognition up to 60% correct in the best-aided condition.[11,12] Thus, it is the case that children with bilateral sensorineural hearing loss—who require full auditory access in the first years of life to achieve auditory, speech, and language development—must have the most severe hearing losses and the poorest speech perception to qualify for implantation.

Despite the restrictive nature of pediatric CI indications, there is considerable evidence to support the expansion of pediatric candidacy. At present, several CI programs are routinely implanting children who may not meet the typical profile, but who are demonstrating significant communication difficulty and/or delayed speech and language development despite appropriate amplification and speech/language intervention. Nonetheless, there are too many children not being referred for CI evaluation because of better than severe-to-profound audiometric thresholds and/or aided speech perception scores exceeding 12% to 30% correct. Thus, the purpose of this article is to describe evidence from the peer-reviewed literature as well as from a new data set to provide data-driven recommendations for expansion of pediatric CI indications.

PEDIATRIC OFF-LABEL COCHLEAR IMPLANTATION

Historically, many CI centers strictly adhered to FDA indications, implanting only children who clearly met those guidelines. However, in recent years, more implant centers have started implanting children outside these guidelines for "off-label" indications. Carlson and colleagues[13] completed a survey of CI surgeons in the United States, and results demonstrated that 78% of the surgeons surveyed (63 of 81) were completing CI surgeries for off-label indications in children and adults. Pertinent to the pediatric population, 43% of surgeons reported implanting children with profound hearing loss less than 12 months of age and 31% implanted children with asymmetric hearing loss whereby at least 1 ear was better than the performance cutoff for age.[13] Consistent with this report, large CI centers in North America have also reported a progressive increase in the number of children being implanted off-label. For example, Na and colleagues[14] reported that 26% of the 389 children implanted at a large Canadian center between 1992 and 2018 had preoperative residual hearing with more than half of the children implanted in the past 2 years having residual hearing. Almost half of these children were reported to have had better than a severe hearing loss in their better ear at the time of diagnosis (43%).[14] Likewise, data from a large academic referral center in the United States also showed a significant increase in the number of children implanted with more residual hearing in recent years.[15]

CHALLENGES OF ASSESSING PEDIATRIC OUTCOMES

Despite a significant increase in the frequency of off-label implantation, obtaining a collection of comprehensive data demonstrating CI benefits in this population is complex and not as straightforward as simply comparing preoperative and postoperative scores on measures of aided speech perception. Unlike adults, children of different ages and developmental abilities will vary in their readiness to complete such assessments with some children being too young to complete any formal measures of speech recognition and older children requiring assessment using different measures appropriate for their age and language level. Assessment of benefit is further complicated by the fact that as a child progresses and ages, assessments previously used become too easy and more difficult material is needed; this can complicate a child's longitudinal assessment. In addition, many centers have historically lacked a formalized protocol for CI candidacy for the pediatric population and/or used monitored-live-voice presentation for assessments, resulting in high across-test variability and significantly inflated speech recognition scores as compared to tests completed using recorded stimuli.[16] In recent years, the pediatric minimum speech test battery (PMSTB[17]) was developed to help standardize the pediatric test protocol. Even with a pediatric test battery now available, it has not been widely implemented in its entirety. In addition, approximately 40% of children with hearing loss have additional disabilities or comorbidities,[18] many of which affect speech and language development, resulting in the need for frequent refinement and modification of assessments used even when the PMSTB is followed.

RESEARCH SUPPORTING EXPANSION OF PEDIATRIC COCHLEAR IMPLANT INDICATIONS

As FDA indications for adult cochlear implantation have evolved, a growing number of CI surgeons are performing off-label CI surgery for children as well. As the frequency of implantation in this population has increased, studies have emerged documenting and quantifying the benefit of cochlear implantation in children who do not meet traditional CI candidacy. Early studies sought to compare performance between children using CIs and children using HAs in an attempt to determine a point at which clinicians could reasonably expect a child to perform better with CIs versus HAs. One such study conducted by Lovett and colleagues[19] demonstrated that children with a 4-frequency pure tone average (PTA; unaided threshold average of 500, 1000, 2000, and 4000 Hz) $\geq$ 80 dB HL in both ears should be considered candidates for implantation given that children with hearing in this range had more than an 80% chance of better speech recognition with CIs vs bilateral HAs. Leigh and colleagues[20] also compared speech recognition results for children receiving CIs before 3 years of age to children using HAs who had moderate, severe, or profound hearing losses. They demonstrated that children with CIs significantly outperformed bilateral HA users who had similar unaided audiograms. Drilling down further, they showed that for children with unaided PTA greater than 60 dB HL, there was a 75% chance that a child would perform better with CIs as compared to bilateral HAs.[20] Their data also suggested that a more conservative referral recommendation—an unaided PTA greater than 82 dB HL—was associated with a 95% chance of achieving significantly higher speech recognition with CIs vs bilateral HAs.[20]

Thus, these data offer clinicians a graded recommendation for audiometric-based candidacy established on relative risk vs reward.

In addition to studies assessing benefit in heterogenous groups of children who do not meet traditional indications for cochlear implantation, other studies have investigated benefit in children with specific configurations and/or degrees of hearing loss. For example, Gratacap and colleagues[21] reviewed CI outcomes for children having (1) residual low-frequency hearing, (2) severe sensorineural hearing loss with poor speech understanding, (3) asymmetric hearing loss, (4) progressive sensorineural hearing loss, and (5) fluctuating sensorineural hearing loss. Their results showed significant improvement on measures of open-set word recognition at 12 months post-implantation in all groups except the low-frequency residual-hearing group. However, this was a small sample (n = 5) with an average implant age of 17 years, and group mean performance still improved by the 24-month point (86%) as compared with the preoperative mean score (79%). Similarly, another study of young children with residual low-frequency hearing and profound high-frequency hearing loss showed significant postoperative improvement, even in cases when hearing was not preserved.[22] Notably, these investigators reported greater improvement in children who were implanted at younger ages.

More recent studies have further described postoperative outcomes in larger populations of nontraditional candidates. Carlson and colleagues[23] described postoperative outcomes for a group of 51 children who had not met labeled indications based on either (1) audiometric thresholds being better than severe-to-profound, and/or (2) aided speech recognition exceeding 30% for preoperative word or sentence recognition. They demonstrated a significant improvement of 63-percentage points in the implanted ear and 40-percentage points in the bimodal condition. Furthermore, every single child achieved benefit in both the implant-only and the bimodal conditions[23] — a rare observation in the literature. Consistent with these results, Park and colleagues[24] reported significant postoperative word recognition benefit for 26 children with a preoperative 4-frequency PTA $\leq$ 75 dB HL. On average, they showed postoperative word recognition scores improved nearly 50-percentage points to a postoperative mean score of 75% as compared with the preoperative time point. A recent retrospective chart review completed by Na and colleagues[14] showed similar postoperative improvement for a group of 34 pediatric CI recipients who had residual hearing before surgery defined as an unaided PTA $\leq$ 90 dB HL in at least 1 ear (median PTA = 77.6 dB HL). They demonstrated significant benefit in monosyllabic word recognition with mean scores improving from 34% (preoperatively) to 90% (postoperatively). They also noted that the proportion of children with preoperative residual hearing who were receiving implants at their center had increased from just 30% of the population in 2004 to 60% in 2018.[14]

There is considerable evidence for the expansion of pediatric CI indications to include children with better than severe-to-profound hearing losses, as children demonstrate significant improvements in speech understanding with CIs as compared with HAs. Despite the growing evidence base, many studies have been limited in scope because of the use of various test metrics necessary to assess a wide range of ages as well as developmental differences in their speech and language skills. This motivated the current study that aimed to investigate benefit of cochlear implantation for children having better than severe-to-profound hearing losses and/or better performance on measures of aided word and sentence recognition than listed by FDA indications. The primary objective of this retrospective review was to assess postoperative word and sentence recognition abilities using the same metrics preimplantation and postimplantation in an updated sample.

METHODS

A retrospective chart review was conducted per institutional review board–approved study (#211178) of pediatric CI recipients being followed for audiological care at a tertiary academic referral center. Medical records of pediatric CI recipients followed at Vanderbilt University Medical Center were reviewed to identify preoperative pure tone thresholds (500, 1000, and 2000 Hz PTA) and preoperative performance on age-appropriate tests of speech recognition. All children included in this study met one or both of the following criteria as originally defined by Carlson and colleagues[23]: (1) greater than 30% correct on an age-appropriate test of aided speech recognition in one or both ears, and/or (2) PTA less than 90 dB HL if younger than 2 years of age or PTA less than 70 dB HL if older than 2 years of age in one or both ears. Children identified with auditory neuropathy spectrum disorder, cochlear nerve deficiency, SSD, or any other developmental conditions expected to negatively impact speech and language development were excluded from review. Children who were not proficient in spoken English were also excluded.

The following information was collected from each participant's medical record: cause of hearing loss, age at time of CI surgery, implant make and model, preoperative unaided PTA in the implanted and nonimplanted ears, and preoperative and postoperative word and sentence recognition scores with HAs or CIs in the ear-specific and bilaterally aided conditions. Word recognition tests included Northwestern University Children's Perception of Speech,[25] Multi-Syllabic Neighborhood Test,[26] Lexical Neighborhood Test,[26] and Consonant Nucleus Consonant.[27] Sentence tests included Hearing in Noise Test for Children, [28] Arizona Biomedical sentences (AzBio[29]), and Pediatric AzBio.[30] Preoperative word and sentence recognition scores and unaided PTAs were obtained from the child's CI candidacy evaluation. In cases for which children were implanted sequentially, data for the second ear were obtained from the most recent assessment before implantation of the second ear. Data for the second implanted ear were only included if the second ear also met inclusion criteria for this study at the time of implantation. Postoperative word and sentence recognition scores were obtained from the most recent audiological evaluation completed 6 or more months postactivation. In some cases, children did not yet have 6-month postactivation scores, and scores obtained sooner than 6 months postactivation were used if postoperative performance already exceeded preoperative performance by the earlier timepoint selected.

Although the chosen assessment measures necessarily varied across patients because of age and language development, preoperative and postoperative comparisons were completed only for children who had been tested using the same recorded measure at both preimplant and postimplant intervals. When preoperative and postoperative comparisons were made for a child having multiple evaluations with the same test metric, the postoperative score selected was the most recent score obtained at least 6 months postoperatively in which no significant equipment or wear time challenges were identified at the time of evaluation.

PARTICIPANTS

Eighty-three patients met inclusion criteria, but 4 of these patients were excluded from final analyses because of diagnoses of intellectual disability and/or developmental delay (n = 3) or lack of postoperative data (n = 1). Analyses were completed on data collected from the medical records of the remaining 79 subjects (44 female subjects). Twenty-nine of the 79 subjects included herein were also included in the authors' previous study.[23] The cause of hearing loss was unknown in over half of the group, and enlarged vestibular aqueduct was the most common cause reported. The distribution of other causes are reported in **Table 1**.

Of the 79 patients, 54 were unilaterally implanted and 25 were bilaterally implanted (4 simultaneously, 21 sequentially). For the 25 bilateral recipients, 21 met study inclusion criteria for 1 ear and the other 4 met criteria in both ears. The mean age of implantation was 8.1 years (range 0.6–18.0 years). Mean unaided PTA was 91.9 dB HL (standard deviation [SD] = 21.1) for all implanted ears and 66.4 dB HL (SD = 21.9) for all nonimplanted ears. All children received the newest technology at the time of implantation with 57.0% of the children having Cochlear devices (n = 45), 27.8% having AB (n = 22), and 15.2% having MED-EL (n = 12).

RESULTS

Fig. 1 displays individual and mean speech recognition scores in quiet and noise for the implanted ear (first column), the bilateral aided condition (second column) preoperatively, as well as for the first postoperative visit (mean CI experience = 2.0 years; range 0.3–7.8 years) and last postoperative visit (mean CI experience = 5.2 years; range 0.3–12.6). Individual data are represented by thin gray lines, and mean data are in bold with error bars representing ±1 standard error of the mean (SEM). Data analysis was completed using repeated-measures analysis of variance with a Geisser-Greenhouse correction for sphericity. Post hoc analyses were completed via Tukey multiple comparisons. Effect sizes were calculated using eta squared values (η^2). The independent variable was the timepoint, and the dependent variable was speech recognition score. Data were analyzed only for participants with both preimplant and postimplant scores for a given measure (see **Fig. 1**).

WORD RECOGNITION

For word recognition in the implant-alone condition, mean scores were 20.6% preoperative, 67.2% first postoperative, and 71.6% second postoperative. Statistical analysis revealed a significant effect of timepoint ($F_{(1.7, 92.3)} = 201.0$, $P<.0001$, $\eta^2 = 0.79$). Post hoc analysis showed a significant difference between both preoperative and first postoperative ($P<.0001$), as well as preoperative and second postoperative ($P<.0001$); however, there was not a difference between the first and second postoperative scores ($P = .18$). For the bilaterally aided condition, mean scores were 56.8% preoperative, 74.6% first postoperative, and 77.6% second postoperative. There was a significant effect of timepoint ($F_{(0.8, 22.3)} = 19.7$, $P = .0003$, $\eta^2 = 0.44$). Post hoc analysis showed a significant difference between both preoperative and first postoperative

Table 1	
Cause for the 79 study participants included in the retrospective review	
Cause	**Number**
Unknown	38
Enlarged vestibular aqueduct	19
Congenital cytomegalovirus	6
Meningitis	5
Prematurity	3
Usher syndrome	3
Connexin	1
Genetic—other	3
Ototoxicity	1

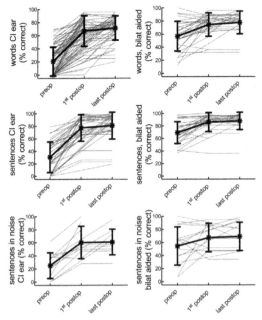

Fig. 1. Individual and mean speech recognition scores for the implanted ear (first column) and bilateral best-aided condition (second column) for word recognition, sentence recognition in quiet, and sentence recognition in noise at +5 dB SNR. Error bars represent ±1 SEM.

(P = .0006), as well as preoperative and second postoperative ($P<$.0001); there was not a difference between the first and second postoperative scores (P = .21).

SENTENCE RECOGNITION IN QUIET

For sentence recognition in quiet in the implant-alone condition, mean scores were 30.6% preoperative, 77.4% first postoperative, and 80.8% second postoperative. Statistical analysis revealed a significant effect of timepoint ($F_{(1.1, 33.1)}$ = 111.8, $P<$.0001, η^2 = 0.78). Post hoc analysis revealed a significant difference between both preoperative and first postoperative ($P<$.0001), preoperative and second postoperative ($P<$.0001), as well as between the first and second postoperative scores (P = .006). For the bilaterally aided condition, mean scores were 69.3% preoperative, 86.1% first postoperative, and 87.9% second postoperative. There was a significant effect of timepoint ($F_{(0.6, 12.3)}$ = 29.5, P = .0006, η^2 = 0.58). Post hoc analysis revealed a significant difference between both preoperative and first postoperative ($P<$.0001), as well as preoperative and second postoperative ($P<$.0001); there was not a significant difference between the first and second postoperative scores (P = .15).

SENTENCE RECOGNITION IN NOISE (+5 dB)

For sentence recognition at a +5 dB signal-to-noise ratio (SNR) in the implant-alone condition, mean scores were 25.2% preoperative, 60.3% first postoperative, and 61.0% second postoperative. Statistical analysis revealed a significant effect of time-point ($F_{(1.9, 15.7)}$ = 22.8, $P<$.0001, η^2 = 0.74). Post hoc analysis revealed a significant difference between both preoperative and first postoperative (P = .0005), as well as preoperative and second postoperative (P = .0009); however, there was not a significant difference between the first and second postoperative scores ($P = .99$). For the bilaterally aided condition, mean scores were 54.6% preoperative, 67.5% first postoperative, and 69.1% second postoperative. There was not a statistically significant effect of timepoint for sentence recognition in noise in the bilaterally aided condition ($F_{(1.1, 12.8)} = 3.2$, $P = .09$, $\eta^2 = 0.21$).

DISCUSSION

Consistent with previous studies, the results from this retrospective review demonstrate that children with better than severe hearing losses and/or greater than 30% aided speech recognition derive significant benefit from cochlear implantation in both the implanted ear and the bilaterally aided conditions. Although the authors did not demonstrate a statistically significant effect of cochlear implantation for sentence recognition in noise in the bilaterally aided condition (see **Fig. 1**, lower righthand panel), over half of those tested demonstrated clinically significant benefit based on 95% confidence interval data for test-retest variability,[30] and the 1 child exhibiting a clinically significant decrement had a documented period of poor device use including a 3-month period of nonuse. Thus, this data set provides further support for expansion of pediatric CI criteria and warrants referrals for children exhibiting auditory and communication difficulties irrespective of whether they meet FDA-labeled indications for implantation.

Despite numerous studies documenting benefits, clinical utilization of cochlear implantation in this population remains poor at many implant centers across the country. More commonly, families of children with greater degrees of residual hearing receive some, but poor, benefit from HAs, and families do not pursue further intervention, often because of fears related to the risk of losing residual hearing and or lack of knowledge that cochlear implantation could provide benefit for their child. Likewise, many pediatric audiologists outside CI centers might not be familiar with outcomes in this population and, thus, are hesitant to refer for a candidacy evaluation. For these reasons, it is common for referring audiologists to rely on the guidelines set forth by traditional FDA indications, which overlook a population of children who would derive significant auditory and communicative benefits. In fact, Park and colleagues[24] showed that for nontraditional pediatric implant recipients, delaying implantation 3 or more years was associated with significantly poorer word recognition outcomes than those implanted within 1 year.

As detailed in the introduction, several methods have been proposed to identify nontraditional pediatric CI candidates for referral. One approach is to refer children with hearing losses exceeding a certain degree, such as that documented by Leigh and colleagues[20] for children with unaided PTA $\geq$ 65 dB HL. Another approach incorporates consideration of both the degree of hearing loss and unaided word recognition abilities. Zwolan and colleagues[31] proposed referring adult recipients for CI evaluation if they demonstrated a best-ear unaided monosyllabic word score $\leq$60% correct and an unaided PTA in the better ear $\geq$60 dB HL. They termed this data-driven recommendation the "60/60 guideline."[31] Although use of this approach has not been assessed in the pediatric population—which could prove difficult for younger children still developing speech and language—there is great potential for applying the 60/60 approach to older children, particularly those with postlingual onset of severe-to-profound hearing loss.

LIMITATIONS

The results of this study are limited by its retrospective nature. Clinical protocols have changed and evolved, resulting in the use of multiple test metrics and test conditions within and across subjects, making it difficult to assess postoperative performance and progress in some patients who would have otherwise met inclusion criteria for this study. Much data were collected before the accessibility of data logging; thus, average device wear time was not available for many of the patients. Although it is possible that poor wear time could have affected outcomes in some cases reported here, it is noteworthy that postoperative speech recognition was significantly higher than preoperative levels for all but 1 measure: sentence recognition in noise in the bilaterally aided condition. Given the correlational relationship between device wear time and speech recognition performance for both adult[32,33] and pediatric[34–36] implant recipients, it is possible that had we been able to account for data logging information, effect sizes would have been larger. Finally, this study did not collect information on aural (re)habilitation completed after implantation.

SUMMARY

The results of this retrospective review are consistent with several previous studies demonstrating significant auditory and speech recognition benefits of cochlear implantation for children who do not meet current FDA labeled indications. Given the critical window for auditory, speech, and language development in children, delays in referral and subsequent implantation could result in significantly poorer auditory outcomes than could have been accomplished if implantation was pursued earlier. There is now considerable evidence in support of revised criteria for pediatric cochlear implantation to include children with better than severe-to-profound sensorineural hearing. Because regulatory changes often lag behind scientific evidence, it is critical that we assess each child individually and refer those who are struggling with auditory speech recognition, age-appropriate speech production, language, and academics.

CLINICS CARE POINTS

- Children with better than severe-to-profound sensorineural hearing loss and those scoring above 30% correct for aided word and sentence recognition demonstrate significant benefit from cochlear implantation.

- Based on evidence in the literature, it is recommended that audiologists and otolaryngologists refer children who have an unaided pure tone average greater than 60 dB HL for a preoperative cochlear implant evaluation.

DISCLOSURE STATEMENT

C. Brown is a consultant for Advanced Bionics. R. Gifford is a consultant for Advanced Bionics, Akouos, Cochlear, and Frequency Therapeutics.

ACKNOWLEDGMENTS

Portions of this data set were presented at the 2017 American Cochlear Implant Alliance (ACIA) meeting, the 2017 Tennessee Academy of Audiology meeting, and the 2021 Sound Foundations Conference. Investigator effort was supported by NIDCD R01 DC017683.

REFERENCES

1. Dettman SJ, Dowell RC, Choo D, et al. Long-term communication outcomes for children receiving cochlear implants younger than 12 months. Otol Neurotol 2016;37(2):e82–95.

2. Wilson B, Dorman M. Interfacing sensors with the nervous system: lessons from the development and success of the cochlear implant. IEEE Sens J 2008;8: 131–47.

3. Roche JP, Hansen MR. On the horizon: cochlear implant technology. Otolaryngol Clin North Am 2015;48(6):1097–116.

4. Houston DM, Stewart J, Moberly A, et al. Word learning in deaf children with cochlear implants: effects of early auditory experience. Dev Sci 2012;15:448–61.

5. Houston DM, Miyamoto RT. Effects of early auditory experience on word learning and speech perception in deaf children with cochlear implants: implications for sensitive periods of language development. Otol Neurotol 2010;31:1248–53.

6. Houston DM, Beer J, Bergeson TR, et al. The ear is connected to the brain: some new directions in the study of children with cochlear implants at Indiana University. J Am Acad Audiol 2012;23(6):446–63.

7. Tomblin JB, Barker BA, Spencer LJ, et al. The effect of age at cochlear implant initial stimulation on expressive language growth in infants and toddlers. J Speech Lang Hear Res 2005;48:853–67.

8. Chweya CM, May MM, DeJong MD, et al. Language and audiological outcomes among infants implanted before 9 and 12 months of age versus older children: a continuum of benefit associated with cochlear implantation at successively younger ages. Otol Neurotol 2021;42(5):686–93.

9. Advanced Bionics. Surgeon's Manual for the HiRes™ Ultra 3D cochlear implant with the HiFocus™ SlimJ and HiFocus™ Mid-Scala Electrodes. Valencia (CA); 2020.

10. MED-EL. Innsbruck (Austria): Mi1250 Synchrony 2 Pin: surgical guide 2020.

11. Cochlear. Sydney (Australia): Nucleus cochlear implants: Physician's Package Insert 2020.

12. CMS. National Coverage Determination for cochlear implantation 100-3 50.3. Centers for Medicare and Medicaid Services; 2005. Available at: https://www.cms.gov/Regulations-and-Guidance/Guidance/Transmittals/Downloads/R42NCD.pdf. Accessed May 31, 2021.

13. Carlson ML, Sladen DS, Gurgel RK, et al. Survey of the American Neurotology Society on Cochlear Implantation: part 1, candidacy assessment and expanding indications. Otol Neurotol 2018;39(1):e12–9.

14. Na E, Toupin-April K, Olds J, et al. Clinical characteristics and outcomes of children with cochlear implants who had residual hearing. Int J Audiol 2021;1–11.

15. Teagle HFB, Park LR, Brown KD, et al. Pediatric cochlear implantation: a quarter century in review. Cochlear Implants Int 2019;20(6):288–98.

16. Uhler K, Biever A, Gifford RH. Method of speech stimulus presentation impacts pediatric speech recognition monitored live voice versus recorded speech. Otol Neurotol 2016;37:e70–4.

17. Uhler K, Warner-Czyz A, Gifford RH. Pediatric minimum speech test battery. J Am Acad Audiol 2017;28(3):232–47.

18. Gallaudet Research Institute. Regional and national summary report of data from the 2013-2014 annual survey of deaf and hard of hearing children and youth. Washington, DC: Gallaudet University; 2015.

19. Lovett R, Vickers D, Summerfield A. Bilateral cochlear implantation for hearing-impaired children: criterion of candidacy derived from an observational study. Ear Hear 2015;36:14–23.

20. Leigh JR, Dettman SJ, Dowell RC. Evidence-based guidelines for recommending cochlear implantation for young children: audiological criteria and optimizing age at implantation. Int J Audiol 2016;55(Suppl 2):S9–18.

21. Gratacap M, Thierry B, Rouillon I. Pediatric cochlear implantation in residual hearing candidates. Ann Otol Rhinol Laryngol 2015;124(6):443–51.
22. Wilson K, Ambler M, Hanvey K, et al. Cochlear implant assessment and candidacy for children with partial hearing. Cochlear Implants Int 2016;17(Suppl 1):66–9.
23. Carlson ML, Sladen DP, Haynes DS, et al. Evidence for the expansion of pediatric cochlear implant candidacy. Otol Neurotol 2015;36(1):43–50.
24. Park L, Perkins E, Woodard J, et al. Delaying cochlear implantation impacts postoperative speech perception of nontraditional pediatric candidates. Audiol Neurootol 2021;26(3):182–7.
25. Elliot LL, Katz DR. Northwestern University children's perception of speech (NU-CHIPS): Technical Manual. Auditec. St. Louis (MO); 1980.
26. Kirk KI, Pisoni DB, Osberger MJ. Lexical effects on spoken word recognition by pediatric cochlear implant users. Ear Hear 1995;16(5):470–81.
27. Peterson GE, Lehiste I. Revised CNC lists for auditory tests. J Speech Hear Disord 1962;27:62–72.
28. Gelnett D, Sumida A, Nilsson M, et al. Development of the hearing-in-noise test for children (HINT-C). Pap Present Annu Meet Am Acad Audiol 1995.
29. Spahr AJ, Dorman MF, Litvak LM, et al. Development and validation of the AzBio sentence lists. Ear Hear 2012;33(1):2–7.
30. Spahr AJ, Dorman MF, Litvak LM, et al. Development and validation of the pediatric AzBio sentence lists. Ear Hear 2014;35(4).
31. Zwolan TA, Schvartz-Leyzac KC, Pleasant T. Development of a 60/60 guideline for referring adults for a traditional cochlear implant candidacy evaluation. Otol Neurotol 2020;41(7):895–900.
32. Schvartz-Leyzac KC, Conrad CA, Zwolan TA. Datalogging statistics and speech recognition during the first year of use in adult cochlear implant recipients. Otol Neurotol 2019;40(7):e686–93.
33. Holder JT, Dwyer NC, Gifford RH. Duration of processor use per day is significantly correlated with speech recognition abilities in adults with cochlear implants. Otol Neurotol 2020;41(2).
34. Wiseman KB, Warner-Czyz A. Inconsistent device use in pediatric cochlear implant users: prevalence and risk factors. Cochlear Implants Int 2018;19:131–41.
35. Easwar V, Sanfilippo J, Papsin B, et al. Impact of consistency in daily device use on speech perception abilities in children with cochlear implants: datalogging evidence. J Am Acad Audiol 2018;29(9):835–46.
36. Busch, T., Vermeulen, A., Langereis, M., et al Cochlear implant data logs predict children's receptive vocabulary. Ear Hear 2020; 41(4):733-746.

Cochlear Implantation for Unilateral Hearing Loss

Anne Morgan Selleck, MD, Kevin D. Brown, MD, PhD, Lisa R. Park, AuD*

KEYWORDS

- Pediatric • Unilateral hearing loss • Cochlear implantation • Single sided deafness

KEY POINTS

- Cochlear implantation in the pediatric severe to profound unilateral hearing loss patient allows for significant improvement in speech recognition in quiet and noise as well as sound localization.
- Outcomes in cochlear implantation in pediatric patients with severe to profound unilateral hearing loss may be impacted by etiology, duration of deafness, and family/patient motivation.
- Additional research is required to determine optimal timing and device choice to allow for maximal outcomes.

INTRODUCTION

Treatment of pediatric unilateral hearing loss (UHL) has changed radically over the past few decades. Before the implementation of newborn hearing screening the average age of diagnosis for UHL was more than 8 years old.[1] As late as the 1970s, the predominant management strategy was reassurance—informing parents UHL has no negative consequences.[2] Research in the 1980s began to shed light on the significance of UHL. Thirty-five percent of children with UHL failed 1 or more grades and up to 60% required special educational services.[3–6] Children with UHL were also noted to have more behavioral issues than their peers with normal hearing, including social withdrawal, aggression, and difficulties with interpersonal and social adjustment.[3,7,8] More recent research has suggested that children with UHL may lag behind in terms of speech and language and cognition as well.[8–10]

Department of Otolaryngology Head and Neck Surgery, The Children's Cochlear Implant Center at UNC, University of North Carolina at Chapel Hill, 501 Fortunes Ridge Drive, Suite A, Durham, NC 27713, USA
* Corresponding author. The Children's Cochlear Implant Center at UNC, 5501 Fortunes Ridge Dr, Suite A, Durham, NC 27713.
E-mail address: lisa_park@med.unc.edu

Otolaryngol Clin N Am 54 (2021) 1193–1203
https://doi.org/10.1016/j.otc.2021.07.002
0030-6665/21/© 2021 Elsevier Inc. All rights reserved.

As part of the Americans with Disabilities Act, the 504 plan ensures that children with UHL receive accommodations to improve access to school curriculums and improve their academic success. Educational support for children with UHL typically involves preferential seating as well as a remote microphone system to minimize the impact of background noise. A hearing aid is another essential tool for the child with UHL who has hearing loss within the range to benefit from traditional amplification. Amplification is usually beneficial for UHL of mild to moderate degree affecting the speech frequencies (500 Hz to 4 kHz).

Children with at least a severe UHL in the speech frequencies may not benefit from traditional amplification. Amplification of greater degrees of hearing loss may not make speech audible, or the perception of speech may be very poor (limited recognition of word and sentences with hearing alone). Children initially benefitting from unilateral amplification may experience progression of hearing loss and no longer benefit.[11] Children with UHL who are unable to benefit from traditional amplification typically have a moderate-to profound loss in the affected ear impacting the speech frequencies (500 Hz to 4 kHz). When hearing loss exceeds these levels, acoustic amplification results in distortion of the speech signal and poor overall speech perception. Children with this degree of UHL and normal hearing in the opposite ear are often referred to as having single-sided deafness (SSD). Treatment options for this population have historically been limited to contralateral routing of signal or bone conduction hearing devices. However, these interventions do not allow for binaural hearing, which is important for auditory development and hearing in dynamic environments.[3,12,13]

There are a number of advantages of hearing from 2 ears, especially in complex listening environments. Stimulation of both auditory pathways allows the brain to take advantage of head shadow, binaural squelch, and binaural summation.[14] These phenomena are best observed when the speech signal and noise are spatially separated, as illustrated in **Fig. 1**. When speech and noise are collocated in front of the child, binaural hearing allows for binaural summation. This improves the determination of loudness and allows for an increase of up to 3 dB in signal-to-noise ratio and up to a 28% improvement in speech perception.[15] When the masker is moved to the better hearing ear, or the left ear in the **Fig. 1** example, the head creates a barrier that results in a decrease in the noise signal on the side of the poorer hearing ear. This is known as the "head shadow effect" and allows for an improved signal-to-noise ratio at the ear contralateral to the noise source. In those with normal hearing bilaterally, the head shadow effect results in improved speech perception as compared with the collocated condition. In the case of SSD, the child would be unable to access the improved signal-to-noise ratio on the poorer hearing side without access to bilateral hearing and the signal is dominated by the noise. Binaural squelch is a more complicated process that allows central auditory pathways to use timing and phase differences in the signal from each ear to improve spatial hearing.

Binaural hearing also allows for sound source localization. Sound arrives with greater amplitude and earlier timing at the ear closest to the signal source. The brain uses these cues for comparison between ears to localize sound, using low frequencies to compare the timing differences and the higher frequencies to compare level differences.[14] These mechanisms are completely dependent on binaural information.

In 2019, the US Food and Drug Administration approved the MED-EL cochlear implant (CI) system for adults and children age 5 years and older with SSD. This is the first CI system approved for this indication in the United States. Cochlear implantation is the first and only treatment option to provide binaural hearing to children with SSD. Positive results are emerging from ongoing clinical trials and retrospective

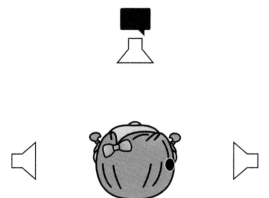

Fig. 1. Spatial hearing in noise. Speech is presented in front (black speech bubble) and the noise signal (white speaker) can be collocated with the speech in front of the listener, directed to the normal hearing (*left*) ear, or directed to the poorer hearing (*right*/implanted) ear. The head shadow effect can be observed here by noting that the implanted ear (*right*) benefits from the physical presence of the head creating an advantageous signal-to-noise ratio (SNR) when noise is directed to the better hearing ear when a CI is in place but not when a CI is off. The head decreases the amount of noise reaching the right ear leading to an improved signal to noise ratio for that ear.

studies have indicated that cochlear implantation in children with SSD is an effective treatment option.[16]

CRITERIA FOR CANDIDACY
Etiology of Hearing Loss

The etiology of the hearing loss has an impact on candidacy. Etiologies of pediatric UHL are more often unknown because there is no comprehensive genetic test battery for UHL, as for bilateral sensorineural hearing loss (SNHL). However, unlike bilateral SNHL, cochlear nerve deficiency (CND) is common in congenital SSD. Therefore imaging, in particular MRI, to directly visualize the eighth nerves, is essential to determine implant candidacy in this population. Other etiologies of significance include congenital cytomegalovirus (CMV) and cochlear malformations. The potential impacts of these conditions are outlined elsewhere in this article.

Cochlear nerve deficiency
CND refers to hypoplasia or aplasia of the cochlear nerve branch of the eighth nerve. CND is the most common etiology for pediatric congenital profound UHL with a reported incidence of 26% to 58%.[17–19] Pediatric CI recipients with bilateral CND have poorer CI outcomes compared with other etiologies. Development of open-set speech perception is not predictable and is often very slow to emerge in this population.[20] The use of CI despite limited benefit in bilateral CND may be warranted because these children otherwise have no access to sound. However, providing children with 1 normal hearing ear with a severely impoverished and distorted auditory signal in the opposite ear is likely to provide a poorer perception of speech. In this situation, the advantages of binaural hearing are not expected, and nonuse is likely. Thus, cochlear implantation is not recommended for individuals with UHL secondary to CND.[17] Ruling

out CND with high resolution 3-dimensional MRI is an essential part of CI candidacy evaluation for children with SSD.

Congenital cytomegalovirus infection

Another common cause of pediatric UHL is congenital CMV infection.[17,19] UHL owing to congenital CMV can be progressive and eventually become bilateral, impacting both treatment of the deaf ear and follow-up of the better hearing ear. With the significant risk of progression, children with SSD owing to congenital CMV should be considered for timely CI.[21]

Additional etiologies

Other potential etiologies for congenital or progressive UHL include inner ear malformations, trauma, meningitis, auditory neuropathy spectrum disorder, sudden idiopathic hearing loss, labyrinthitis, and ototoxic medications, as well as neurologic, syndromic, and other unknown causes. In regard to inner ear malformations, the most common is an incomplete partition type 2 followed by a narrowed internal auditory canal and enlarged vestibular aqueduct.[22] Although children with incomplete partition type 2 and/or an enlarged vestibular aqueduct can perform as well as children with normal cochleae, severely malformed cochlea may also limit functional outcomes and therefore are not suited for implantation in children with SSD.[23]

Duration of Deafness

Early implantation, thus minimizing the period of auditory deprivation, is associated with better speech perception of children with bilateral SNHL who receive CIs. Evidence in the SSD population also supports an optimal window for intervention. Those with SSD have the unique issue of aural preference syndrome, a reorganization of the central auditory pathways for the dominant hearing ear.[24] To prevent this central preference and to allow for a good binaural hearing, outcome data suggest that implantation should be within the first 5 years of life. Evidence supporting this window includes histopathology and MRI studies examining central auditory pathway myelination and plasticity.[25–27] Case studies of cortical evoked potential changes after CI in children with SSD have also supported these findings by noting improvements in cortical reorganization in children with less than 5 years of deafness.[28,29]

Some retrospective case series of children with congenital SSD have demonstrated poorer speech perception outcomes when the duration of deafness is prolonged.[20,30,31] The authors of these works recommend implantation at less than 3 or 4 years of age to encourage maximal CI outcomes in children with SSD.[30] However, there are case reports indicating positive CI outcomes in cases of prolonged congenital SSD.[32] Given the small number of published reports involving CI in children with SSD, and variables such as programming techniques, electrode length, consistency of device use, and postimplant habilitation, which may impact outcomes, the age range within which significant benefit may still occur remains undefined.

Family and Patient Factors

Parents of young children with SSD are less likely to pursue CI than those with children with bilateral SNHL.[33] The decision-making process is fundamentally different because children with SSD develop spoken language and learning delays may not be apparent until they reach elementary school. Therefore, the benefits of binaural hearing, and not mode of communication, are weighed against the risk of surgery, the use of an external device, and the need for lifelong audiologic care.

For families that pursue CI, their commitment to ensure their child consistently use the device is critical to performance.[34,35] Unlike children with bilateral CIs, those with

SSD may struggle, but can still communicate with spoken language without their device. Therefore, the need for consistent device use may not be as clear or compelling to the family, and the risk of device nonuse is increased.

Older children with SSD have been reported to be at increased risk to become nonusers.[31,36] Therefore, it is important that older children be involved in the decision-making process and be willing to commit to device use.

OBSERVATIONAL OUTCOMES OF COCHLEAR IMPLANTATION FOR SINGLE-SIDED DEAFNESS
Word Recognition in Quiet

Unlike other hearing interventions, cochlear implantation allows for speech perception in the ear with SSD. Overall, the literature demonstrates the potential of a CI to improve word recognition. Implanted children with SSD, particularly those with a shorter duration of unilateral deafness, demonstrate a significant improvement in their word recognition scores in the CI-only condition, with scores as high as 90%.[17,31,35–38] Children with longer durations of deafness, ranging from 4 to 13 years often have poorer word recognition outcomes.[31,35,36] However, isolated word recognition is not a measure of the real-world impact of CI on the daily lives of children with SSD. These impacts would include listening effort, localization of sound, hearing in noise, and academic and social skills.

Sound Source Localization

One of the principal benefits of binaural hearing is sound source localization. Studies have demonstrated a significant improvement in sound localization in the "CI on" condition in the majority of CI recipients with SSD.[17,32,39] Localization abilities tend to correlate with speech perception outcomes, although there have been some patients who demonstrate improvement in sound localization with limited or no speech perception in quiet in the implanted ear.[17,35] Improved sound localization has been seen as early as 1 month after CI activation with benefit maintained long term.[35] Parental surveys of auditory behavior also have demonstrated subjective improvement in localization and spatial hearing.[17,32]

Speech Perception in Noise

In children, the ability to hear in dynamic listening environments, which include varying degrees of background noise, is paramount to learning. Speech perception testing in noise is important because it permits the measurement of a binaural advantage, particularly when speech and noise are separated in their presentation (**Fig. 1**). Separating the signals allows for the evaluation of binaural summation, binaural squelch, and the head shadow advantage. Binaural summation can be measured by comparing speech perception scores with unilateral versus bilateral hearing when speech and noise are collocated in front of the listener. Studies have demonstrated summation benefits in the collocated condition among children with UHL and CI.[30,35,40,41] Similarly, head shadow benefit can be calculated by comparison of unilateral versus bilateral conditions (CI on vs CI off) when the speech signal is in front of the listener and the noise is directed to the better hearing ear. Children with SSD who use a CI have shown evidence of benefit from head shadow.[17,32,37,40,41] Benefit from the squelch effect can be measured with by comparing unilateral and bilateral speech perception outcomes obtained with speech in front of the listener and noise at the poorer hearing ear. Evidence of squelch is mixed in adult studies, with some noting no benefit in CI users with SSD[42,43] and others noting benefit after 1 or more years of CI use.[42–45] Small amounts of binaural squelch benefit may be measurable in some children with SSD who use CI for more than 1 year.[41]

Some studies of speech perception in noise support duration of deafness and etiology as influencing outcome, whereas others do not.[17,30,32,40] Interestingly, similar to localization abilities, some children with SSD and CI who do not have measurable open set word recognition still report subjective improvement in hearing in noise.[35] In general, a comparison of speech perception in spatially separated speech and noise with CI on versus CI off has demonstrated that a CI does not interfere with overall speech understanding, regardless of performance with the CI alone, alleviating concerns regarding binaural interference.[36]

Device Use

Device use is critical to improvement and benefit from a CI. This point has been demonstrated clearly in individuals with bilateral SNHL. Most pediatric SSD CI studies report full time use in more than 75% of children with a minority of recipients as nonusers.[9,17,30,31,36,40] Reasons cited for device nonuse include a subjective lack of improvement with device use, nonauditory stimulation, poor family support, stigmatization and negative attention as a result of device use, and older implantation age.[17,36] Counseling is an important tool to establish realistic expectations and encourage full-time use.

Speech and Language Development

Although children with SSD develop spoken language, there is evidence of impact upon language and academics in these children in comparison to children with normal hearing.[9] One longitudinal study compared 6 children with congenital SSD, implanted between ages 8 and 26 months, with normal hearing peers and with unimplanted children with congenital SSD.[9] Language comprehension, expressive vocabulary, morphosyntactic knowledge, and cognitive skills were examined. The SSD CI group performed similarly to the normal hearing group, whereas approximately 50% of the nonimplanted children with SSD performed lower than the normal hearing group in each category.[9] This study supports the concept that CI may enable development of language skills and cognitive milestones in children with SSD equivalent to normal hearing children.

SUBJECTIVE OUTCOMES OF COCHLEAR IMPLANTATION FOR SINGLE-SIDED DEAFNESS
Speech, Spatial, and Qualities of Hearing Scale

The Speech, Spatial, and Qualities of Hearing Scale is a self-reported measure with a modified version for parental report to evaluate subjective hearing abilities in 3 separate areas sensitive to binaural hearing.[46] Studies of the impact of CI on children with SSD have demonstrated consistent improvement in all 3 areas evaluated by the Speech, Spatial, and Qualities of Hearing Scale survey, with the greatest improvement in spatial hearing.[17,31,39,40,47] High performers tend to show correlation between Speech, Spatial, and Qualities of Hearing Scale scores and behavioral CI measures including word recognition scores, sound localization, and daily CI use.[17]

Tinnitus

Tinnitus, one of the original reasons for cochlear implantation in adults with SSD, has also been examined in the pediatric population. The incidence of tinnitus in children with a CI is estimated to be 38%.[48] Zeitler and colleagues[38] reported on the impact of CI on tinnitus in children with SSD. The authors found that 50% experienced partial suppression and 50% complete resolution while using a CI.[38]

Academic and Personal Performance

SSD also impacts children's academic and personal well-being. In 1 study, a parental survey on a nonvalidated questionnaire demonstrated positive behavior change attributed to CI was noted by parents of one-half of the implanted children, as well as improvement in mental serenity and tranquility in 28%.[40] Improvement in peer interactions after implantation has also been reported on parental survey.[32] Children with SSD with little to no speech perception in quiet with the CI side only have also reported improvement in quality of life as well as academic performance both on parental and child report, likely related to the improvements still noted in sound localization as well as speech perception in noise.[35]

Child and Family Satisfaction

Parental and child satisfaction after implantation has been reported to be favorable in several studies. One study reported that 84.2% of parents would select cochlear implantation again if given the choice.[40] Another study reported that all children in the cohort were very satisfied with their decision to undergo implantation.[32]

DEVICE CONSIDERATIONS

There are theoretic reasons why implantation of longer electrodes may be beneficial for implanted patients, particularly those with SSD. Longer electrode arrays, which extend into the apex of the cochlea, allow for improved frequency–place matching when programming a CI by representing a larger range of frequencies in the cochlea.[49,50] Frequency–place matching refers to stimulation of the cochlea at sites that are appropriate for the desired frequency based on the normal tonotopic organization of the cochlea. The more accurate frequency–place matching, the more closely electric hearing may approximate hearing in the normal ear, thereby hastening the integration of binaural hearing of 2 different types of auditory stimulation.[51] This factor may decrease the brain remapping necessary for the integration of electric and acoustic hearing. Rapid integration soon after device activation may aid in achieving device acceptance and consistent use, which may be especially advantageous in children. Additionally, longer electrode arrays have also been shown to improve spatial hearing.[52] Studies of the impact of frequency–place mapping specifically on SSD outcomes are needed. However, in light of current knowledge, longer electrode length should be a consideration when implanting children with SSD.

FUTURE DIRECTIONS

The current pediatric SSD and CI literature primarily consists of retrospective reviews of small series of CI recipients. Given the significant heterogeneity of the population in terms of length of deafness, etiology, cognition, and CI device/electrode, well-designed prospective clinical trials are needed to understand best practices to optimize outcome, potential benefits and range of outcome.

SUMMARY

Cochlear implantation in the pediatric patient with SSD can result in significant objective improvements in speech perception in the deafened ear, speech recognition in noise, and localization, as well as subjective improvements in tinnitus, speech and language development and academic performance. Eligible patients should have a normal cochlear nerve. Candidacy considerations should include etiology of deafness including risk of future loss in the normal hearing ear, duration of deafness, and the child and family's commitment to cochlear implantation.

CLINICS CARE POINTS

- Improvements that can be expected from cochlear implantation in the child with SSD include better speech perception in quiet and noise, sound localization, speech and language development, and quality of life.

- Children with SSD owing to CND are not candidates for CI. Nerve deficiency should be evaluated by high resolution 3-dimensional MRI of the internal auditory canals.

- CI for SSD is of special consideration in children with history of congenital CMV or cochlear malformation that places the child's one normal hearing ear at risk for future hearing loss.

- The duration of deafness, with shorter being more favorable, and patient and family motivation should be considered in the decision for implantation.

DISCLOSURE

Dr Kevin Brown is on the MED-EL Corporation Surgical Advisory board. Dr Lisa Park receives research grant support provided to her university by MED-EL Corporation.

REFERENCES

1. Brookhouser PE, Worthington DW, Kelly WJ. Unilateral hearing loss in children. Laryngoscope 1991;101:1264–72.
2. Northern J, Downs M. Hearing in children. 2nd edition. Baltimore, MD: Williams & Wilkins; 1978. p. 143.
3. Bess FH, Tharpe AM. Unilateral hearing impairment in children. Pediatrics 1984; 74:206–16.
4. Oyler RF, Oyler AL, Matkin ND. Unilateral hearing loss: demographics and educational impact. Lang Sp Hear Serv Schools 1988;19:201–10.
5. Bovo R, Martini A, Angoletto M, et al. Auditory and academic performance of children with unilateral hearing loss. Scand Audiol Suppl 1998;30:71–4.
6. Jensen JH, Børre S, Johansen PA. Unilateral sensorineural hearing loss in children: cognitive abilities with respect to right/left differences. Br J Audiol 1989; 23:215–20.
7. Stein D. Psychosocial characteristics of school-age children with unilateral hearing losses. J Acad Rehabil Audiol 1983;16:12–22.
8. Lieu JEC. Unilateral hearing loss in children: speech-language and school performance. B-ENT 2013;21:107–15.
9. Sangen A, Dierckx A, Boudewyns A, et al. Longitudinal linguistic outcomes of toddlers with congenital single-sided deafness – six with and twelve without cochlear implant and nineteen normal hearing peers. Clin Otolaryngol 2019;44: 671–6.
10. Sangen A, Royackers L, Desloovere C, et al. Single sided deafness affects language and auditory development – a case-control study. Clin Otolaryngol 2017;42(5):979–87.
11. Lieu JEC. Permanent unilateral hearing loss (UHL) and childhood development. Curr Otorhinolaryngol Rep 2018;6:74–81.

12. Lin LM, Bowditch S, Anderson MJ, et al. Amplification in the rehabilitation of unilateral deafness: speech in noise and directional hearing effects with bone-anchored hearing and contralateral routing of signal amplification. Otol Neurotol 2006;27:172–82.
13. Niparko JK, Cox KM, Lustig LR. Comparison of the bone anchored hearing aid implantable hearing device with contralateral routing of offside signal amplification in the rehabilitation of unilateral deafness. Otol Neurotol 2003;24:73–8.
14. Akeroyd MA. The psychoacoustics of binaural hearing. Int J Audiol 2006;45(S1): S25–33.
15. Litovsky R, Parkinson A, Arcaroli J, et al. Simultaneous bilateral cochlear implantation in adults: a multicenter clinical study. Ear Hear 2006;27(6):714–31.
16. Benchetrit L, Ronner E, Anne S, et al. Cochlear implantation in children with single-sided deafness: a systematic review and meta-analysis. JAMA Otolaryngol Head Neck Surg 2021;147(1):58–69.
17. Arndt S, Prosse S, Laszig R, et al. Cochlear implantation in children with single-sided deafness: does aetiology and duration of deafness matter? Audiol Neurotol 2015;20(S1):21–30.
18. van Wieringen A, Boudewyns A, Sangen A, et al. Unilateral congenital hearing loss in children: challenges and potentials. Hear Res 2019;372:29–41.
19. Usami S, Kitoh R, Moteki H, et al. Etiology of single-sided deafness and asymmetrical hearing loss. Acta Otolaryngol 2017;S565:S2–7.
20. Young NM, Kim FM, Ryan ME, et al. Pediatric cochlear implantation of children with eighth nerve deficiency. Int J Pediatr Otorhinolaryngol 2012;1442–8.
21. Gross SD, Ross DS, Dollard SC. Congenital cytomegalovirus infection as a cause of permanent bilateral hearing loss: a quantitative assessment. J Clin Virol 2008; 41(2):57–62.
22. Song J-J, Choi HG, Oh SH, et al. Unilateral sensorineural hearing loss in children: the importance of temporal bone computed tomography and audiometric follow-up. Otol Neurotol 2009;30:604–8.
23. Buchman CA, Copeland BJ, Yu KK, et al. Cochlear implantation in children with congenital inner ear malformations. Laryngoscope 2004;114:309–16.
24. Kral A, Hubka P, Heid S, et al. Single-sided deafness leads to unilateral aural preference within an early sensitive period. Brain 2013;136:180–93.
25. Su P, Kuan CC, Kaga K, et al. Myelination progression in language-correlated regions in brain of normal children determined by quantitative MRI assessment. Int J Pediatr Otorhinolaryngol 2008;72(12):1751–63.
26. Kinney HC, Brody BA, Kloman AS, et al. Sequence of central nervous system myelination in human infancy. II. Patterns of myelination in autopsied infants. J Neuropathol Exp Neurol 1988;47(3):217–34.
27. Sharma A, Dorman MF, Spahr AJ. A sensitive period for the development of the central auditory system in children with cochlear implants: implications for age of implantation. Ear Hear 2002;23:532–9.
28. Sharma A, Glick H, Campbell J, et al. Cortical plasticity and re-organization in pediatric single-sided deafness pre- and post- cochlear implantation: a case study. Otol Neurotol 2016;37(2):e26–34.
29. Polonenko M, Gordon K, Cushing S, et al. Cortical organization restored by cochlear implantation in young children with single sided deafness. Scientific Rep 2017;7(1):1–8.
30. Tavora-Vieira D, Rajan GP, Van de Heyning P, et al. Evaluating the long-term hearing outcomes of cochlear implant users with single-sided deafness. Otol Neurotol 2019;40:e575–80.

31. Beck RL, Aschendorff A, Hassepass F, et al. Cochlear implantation in children with congenital unilateral deafness: a case series. Otol Neurotol 2017;38:e570–6.

32. Ehrmann-Mueller D, Kurz A, Kuehn H, et al. Usefulness of cochlear implantation in children with single sided deafness. Int J Pediatr Otorhinolaryngol 2020;130: 109808.

33. Cushing SL, Gordon KA, Sokolov M, et al. Etiology and therapy indication for cochlear implantation in children with single-sided deafness. HNO 2019;67: 750–9.

34. Easwar V, Sanfilippo J, Papsin B, et al. Impact of consistency in daily device use on speech perception abilities in children with cochlear implants: datalogging evidence. J Am Acad Audiol 2018;29:835–46.

35. Rahne T, Plontke SK. Functional result after cochlear implantation in children and adults with single-sided deafness. Otol Neurotol 2016;37:e332–40.

36. Deep NL, Gordon SA, Shapiro WH, et al. Cochlear implantation in children with single-sided deafness. Laryngoscope 2021;131:e271–7.

37. Sladen DP, Frisch CD, Carlson ML, et al. Cochlear implantation for single-sided deafness: a multicenter study. Laryngoscope 2017;127:223–8.

38. Zeitler DM, Sladen DP, DeJong MD, et al. Cochlear implantation for single-sided deafness in children and adolescents. Int J Pediatr Otorhinolaryngol 2019;118: 128–33.

39. Ramos MÁ, Borkoski-Barreiro SA, Falcón González JC, et al. Single-sided deafness and cochlear implantation in congenital and acquired hearing loss in children. Clin Otolaryngol 2019;44:138–43.

40. Thomas JP, Neumann K, Dazert S, et al. Cochlear implantation in children with congenital single-sided deafness. Otol Neurotol 2017;38:496–503.

41. Park LR, Dillon MT, Buss E, et al. Spatial release from masking in pediatric cochlear implant recipients with single-sided deafness. Am J Audiol 2021; 30(2):443–51.

42. Buss E, Dillon MT, Rooth MA, et al. Effects of cochlear implantation on binaural hearing in adults with unilateral hearing loss. Trends Hearing 2018;22:1–15.

43. Mertens G, De Bodt M, Van De Heyning P. Evaluation of long-term cochlear implant use in subjects with acquired unilateral profound hearing loss: focus on binaural auditory outcomes. Ear Hear 2017;38(1):117–25.

44. Friedmann DR, Ahmed OH, McMenomey SO, et al. Single-sided deafness cochlear implantation: candidacy, evaluation, and outcomes in children and adults. Otol Neurotol 2016;37(2):e154–60.

45. Grossmann W, Brill S, Moeltner A, et al. Cochlear implantation improves spatial release from masking and restores localization abilities in single-sided deaf patients. Otol Neurotol 2016;37(6):658–64.

46. Gatehouse S, Noble W. The Speech, Spatial and Qualities of hearing scale (SSQ). Int J Audiol 2004;43(2):85–99.

47. Hassepass F, Aschendorff A, Wesarg T, et al. Unilateral deafness in children: audiologic and subjective assessment of hearing ability after cochlear implantation. Otol Neurotol 2012;34:53–60.

48. Chada NK, Gordon KA, James AL, et al. Tinnitus is prevalent in children with cochlear implants. Int J Pediatr Otorhinolaryngol 2009;73:671–5.

49. Hochmair I, Hochmair E, Nopp P, et al. Deep electrode insertion and sound coding in cochlear implants. Hear Res 2015;322:14–23.

50. Svirsky MA, Talavage TM, Sinha S, et al. Gradual adaptation to auditory frequency mismatch. Hear Res 2015;322:163–70.

51. Dillon MT, Buss E, Rooth MA, et al. Low-frequency pitch perception in cochlear implant recipients with normal hearing in the contralateral ear. J Speech Lang Hear Res 2019;62(8):2860–71.
52. Zhou X, Li H, Yuan W, et al. Effects of insertion depth on spatial speech perception in noise for simulations of cochlear implants and single-sided deafness. Int J Audiol 2017;56(SUP2):S41–8.

Bone Conduction
Benefits and Limitations of Surgical and Nonsurgical Devices

Hillary Snapp, AuD, PhD

KEYWORDS

- Baha • Binaural hearing • Bone conduction device • Bone conduction implant
- Conductive hearing loss • Unilateral hearing loss • Transcutaneous

KEY POINTS

- Current evidence supports early intervention with BCDs to improve outcomes in children with conductive and mixed hearing loss.
- Direct drive implant systems provide significantly improved hearing outcomes over passive transcutaneous stimulation.
- Bilateral fitting of BCDs consistently demonstrates improved performance over unilateral fitting in children with bilateral hearing impairment.

INTRODUCTION

Early identification and rehabilitation of childhood hearing loss (HL) is essential in mitigating the potential negative consequences of HL on overall development. Evidence demonstrates that early intervention promotes speech and language development and has positive effects on academic outcomes and social-emotional development.[1] Effective intervention can prove challenging in cases of congenital HL or early onset of other forms of irresolvable hearing conditions that cannot be readily managed through medical intervention or traditional hearing aids. The most common examples of such challenging conditions include congenital anomalies of the external and/or middle ear associated with partial or complete closure of the external canal. Furthermore, when combined with microtia or a malformed pinna, traditional hearing aids cannot be retained. In such cases, sound can be transmitted via bone conduction (BC) directly to the healthy cochlea, thus bypassing any conductive component. BC devices (BCDs) have become a well-accepted treatment for managing childhood conductive HL (CHL) and mixed HL, which can also accompany chronic otitis media, chronic otitis externa, cholesteatoma, or ossicular abnormalities.[2,3] It is also possible to use BCDs to reroute signals from the side of a deafened ear to the better hearing ear as in the

Department of Otolaryngology, University of Miami, 1120 Northwest 14th Street, 5th Floor, Miami, FL 33136, USA
E-mail address: hsnapp@med.miami.edu

Otolaryngol Clin N Am 54 (2021) 1205–1217
https://doi.org/10.1016/j.otc.2021.07.015

case of unilateral severe to profound sensorineural HL. Although the vast majority of BCD users experience improved hearing outcome and report improved quality of life, technological and design limitations have prevented the widespread use and adoption of these devices, particularly in the pediatric population.[2–6] There have been considerable technological advancements of BCDs since their first introduction in 1977, with the field of BC hearing rapidly evolving.[7] Although BCDs can be used in children with recurrent and/or fluctuating CHL, this review aims to present and discuss the clinical use, benefits, and limitations of BCDs in the management of permanent childhood HL.

BONE CONDUCTION HEARING

Hearing by way of BC relies on the propagation of sound waves through the bones of the skull to the cochlea. Sound transmission by BC is influenced by a complex combination of mechanisms including the passive movement of the ossicles and inner ear fluids that dominates at low frequencies, sound radiation in the external and middle ear spaces, and compression mechanics.[8–10] BC is an efficient means of transmitting sound to the cochlea and evokes similar responses to sound as does air conduction.[11,12] However, the sound transmission properties will change some perceptual aspects of the sound.

Unlike air-conducted stimuli, both cochleae are stimulated when a sound is transmitted via BC. In addition, stimulation of the skull results in unique interaural timing and level differences between the cochleae that can vary with the location of the stimulation point. That is, the skull has resonances and antiresonances that can affect sound transmission and the frequency response of the skull will vary depending on the stimulation point. BC signal attenuation by the skull at the contralateral cochlea can be significant. Therefore, the ear ipsilateral to the device will have lower (better) thresholds than the ear contralateral to the device and these level differences vary by frequency. Reduction of transmission to the contralateral ear is greater for high- than for low-frequency sounds, which may impact speech recognition.[9,13,14] In addition, interaural time delays for BC stimuli are relatively short compared with those for air-conducted stimuli.[9,15] Differences in size, shape, and thickness of the skull can also affect transmission of the BC signal to the cochlea. These differences influence sound perception by individuals relying on BC to hear.

Bone Conduction Hearing in Children

How the differences in hearing with air conduction versus BC affect the developing auditory system is not entirely understood. Sensitivity to bone-conducted sound has been shown to be better in infants than in older children and adults, with the greatest sensitivity occurring in the low frequencies.[16,17] This observation is likely due to the smaller size and thinner bone of the skull during early childhood. In addition, the presence of fontanelles in early life changes the vibratory properties of the skull. Thus, although thresholds to sound from a BCD on the ipsilateral side are better in children than adults, reduction of sound to the contralateral ear is much greater when the fontanelles are open, resulting in poorer thresholds.[17,18] This reduction in sound transmission due to open fontanelles is between 10 and 30 dB.[17]

Fitting BCDs in children brings additional challenges because they may not be able to report distortions or issues with loudness tolerance. It is not uncommon for adults with CHL to experience reduced loudness tolerance, especially to their own voice and low-frequency sounds when stimulated by a BCD. Patients with this complaint may require an adaptation period and reduction in low-frequency gain of the BCD in such cases; overamplification of low frequencies might interfere with audibility of higher-frequency sounds. Studies on the effects of different BC fitting strategies on speech and language development in children are lacking.

BONE CONDUCTION DEVICES

The most common indication for BCDs in childhood is aural atresia. BCDs can be nonsurgical by placing an externally worn sound processor and transducer on the mastoid region. Alternatively, a surgically implanted osseointegrated device can be coupled to an external sound processor. Currently available systems in the United States are presented in **Table 1**.

Nonsurgical Transcutaneous Bone Conduction Devices

Nonsurgical BCDs are essential to the management of children too young for, or who are poor candidates for, a surgically implanted BCD. Nonsurgical BCDs are often the only treatment option for children unable to wear conventional hearing aids, such as those with aural atresia. Nonsurgical BCDs are typically worn over the mastoid region coupled via a headband (**Fig. 1**). A more recent alternative is to couple the BCD to a medical-grade adhesive pad affixed to the skin in the postauricular area.[19] Although from a sound transmission standpoint BCD placement over the mastoid is optimal, wearing them in that location is not practical for infants and young children unable to sit and independently hold up their head. Instead, consistent early access to sound should be prioritized by placing the BCD anywhere between the 2 mastoids along the frontal bone. As the child develops head control and spends more time upright, the processor can be moved to the mastoid position to provide optimal stimulation. Other limitations of nonsurgical BCDs include discomfort with long wear times either from the head band or from chronic adhesive use.

Nonsurgical BCDs rely on transcutaneous stimulation where sound is transmitted through vibration of intact skin to the underlying skull; this results in less-efficient sound transmission than that obtained with direct stimulation of the bone. The presence of skin and underlying soft tissue dampens signal transmission, which can result in a loss of more than 20 dB, with higher-frequency sound transmission being more affected.[20–22] Poor or reduced access to high-frequency speech cues with transcutaneous stimulation may limit the benefits of BCDs and negatively impact speech and language development.[23,24]

Although nonsurgical transcutaneous BCDs are essential in providing early intervention options for children with CHL and mixed HL, issues with mechanical feedback and device placement can prove difficult for young children and parents to manage. Counseling about management of these practical concerns is important for successful and consistent device use. To achieve optimal hearing, the fitting range and device output must be considered. There are several BCDs now available, each with different gain characteristics that can significantly influence the dynamic range of speech available to the child.[25] Because of signal attenuation associated with nonsurgical transcutaneous BCDs, use of higher-gain devices is recommended in early and school-aged children.[26] In cases of mixed HL in which the BC hearing is not within the normal range, choice of the device and settings to optimize gain and output of the BCD is even more critical.

Surgically implanted bone conduction devices

Percutaneous devices
Percutaneous BC implants (see **Fig. 1**) consist of a detachable external sound processor coupled by an abutment that penetrates the skin and is connected to an

Table 1
Bone conduction device characteristics and specifications

	Stimulation	Coupling	Device, Manufacturer	FDA Approved[a] MRI	FDA Approved[a] Age	FDA Approved[a] Fit Range
Nonsurgical	Passive/transcutaneous	Headband	Baha, Cochlear Americas	N/A	N/A	Standard 45 dB SNHL, up to 65 dB SNHL with power processors[b]
			Ponto, Oticon Medical			Standard 45 dB SNHL, up to 65 dB SNHL with power processors[b]
		Adhesive	ADHEAR, MED-EL			Up to 25 dB SNHL
			ADHEAR, MED-EL			Up to 25 dB SNHL
Surgical	Passive/transcutaneous	Magnet	Attract, Cochlear Americas	Up to 1.5 T	≥5 y	Standard 45 dB SNHL, up to 65 dB SNHL with power processors[b]
			Medtronic Alpha 2 MPO ePlus[d]	Up to 3 T[c]	≥5 y	Up to 45 dB SNHL
	Direct	Percutaneous implant	Baha Connect, Cochlear Americas	Up to 3 T	≥5 y	Standard 45 dB SNHL, up to 65 dB SNHL with power processors[b]
			Ponto, Oticon Medical	Up to 3 T	≥5 y	Standard 45 dB SNHL, up to 65 dB SNHL with power processors[b]
	Direct/active transcutaneous	Magnet	BONEBRIDGE, MED-EL	Up to 1.5 T	≥12 y	Up to 45 dB SNHL
			OSIA, Cochlear Americas	Up to 1.5 T with magnet removed	≥12 y	Up to 55 dB SNHL

Abbreviations: SNHL, sensorineural hearing loss.
[a] All reported FDA approvals are current as June 2021.
[b] Systems consist of a range of compatible sound processors with varying force output levels allowing for a broader fit range.
[c] Magnet not removable.
[d] Implant (Sophono Alpha 2) no longer commercially available, only processor is available.

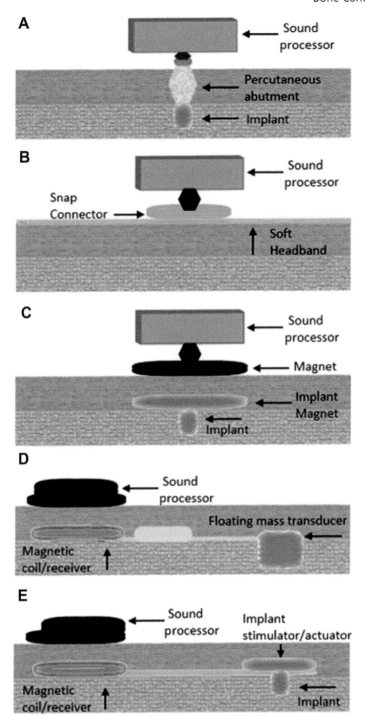

Fig. 1. Bone conduction devices: (*A*) direct drive osseointegrated implant with percutaneous abutment, (*B*) passive transcutaneous nonsurgical BCD on a soft headband, (*C*) passive transcutaneous implant system using magnetic coupling, (*D*) active direct drive implant using a floating mass transducer, (*E*) active direct drive implant using a piezoelectric stimulator with an osseointegrated implant.

osseointegrated implant in the temporal bone. The direct coupling of the implant to the temporal bone allows for highly efficient transmission of bone-conducted sound to the cochlea. Despite this, percutaneous BCD use is limited in the pediatric population because of increased occurrence of skin problems at the abutment, cosmetic concerns, and increased risk of failure of osseointegration, especially in young children.[27,28] Percutaneous implants also require daily care and lifelong management. Skin complications occur anywhere from 5% to 26% in children.[2,27–30] Although skin problems are often minor, in some cases soft tissue overgrowth requires surgical debridement.

Percutaneous implant stability relies on successful osseointegration of the implant fixture. Failure of osseointegration is most common during the first 4 years of life when bone is thin and rapidly growing.[31] For this reason, percutaneous BCD implants are generally reserved for children aged 5 years and older where bone has likely matured to at least 2.5 mm thickness.[26] Osseointegration failure rate is usually 3% to 6% but has been reported as high as 14%.[29,30,32] For these reasons, it is standard practice to delay fitting of the external processor in children by at least 3 months after surgery. Longer osseointegration periods should be considered in children at increased risk of osseointegration failure, such as those with craniofacial anomalies.[26,33,34] As children grow, they are also at increased risk for implant loss due to trauma.[4,30,33] The marked changes in soft tissue during childhood growth are associated with skin problems requiring surgical debridement and higher rates of implant loss.[4,30,33]

Transcutaneous devices. Transcutaneous BCD implants avoid the complications that come with skin-penetrating percutaneous implants. Early transcutaneous BCDs rely on passive stimulation by magnetic coupling of the internal and external components. The external speech processor transmits acoustic vibration through intact skin and soft tissue to the internal device (see **Table 1**). In terms of effectiveness of sound transmission, this technology is comparable to nonsurgical transcutaneous BCDs and thereby subject to similar reductions in gain due to energy absorption by skin and soft tissue.

Active transcutaneous devices. Active transcutaneous implantable BCDs were developed to provide the superior hearing of percutaneous BCD implants while still offering the benefits of transcutaneous coupling and avoiding the problems associated with skin penetration.[24,35–37] First introduced in 2012, active transcutaneous direct-drive BCD implants consist of an external sound processor magnetically coupled to the surgical implant. The processor sends a signal through the intact skin to the implant, which contains a receiver and a transducer.[38] Unlike passive transcutaneous BCD implants, the signal is converted to vibration within the surgical implant. This conversion enables bone to be directly stimulated while leaving skin intact and without subjecting skin to vibration.[36,39–43] The result is that active BCD implants avoid sound attenuation by intact skin. In addition, magnet strength needed for coupling with this arrangement is typically reduced,[44] which lessens the risk of skin irritation.

Various active transcutaneous BCD implants have been developed with differences in implant design, device output, surgical approach, and surgical candidacy (see **Table 1**).[36,45,46] All active transcutaneous BCD implants still require internal and external magnets to couple the external processor and the surgical implant. The 2 systems available in the United States transform the signal sent to the implant across intact skin into mechanical vibration by different methods. The BONEBRIDGE (MED-EL, Durham, NC, USA) uses an electromagnetic floating mass transducer, and the Osia (Cochlear Americas, Denver, CO, USA) uses a piezoelectric transducer.

The piezoelectric transducer is reported to have improved high-frequency gain over passive transcutaneous BCD implants and percutaneous BCD implants, resulting in improved speech perception.[47] As providing access to high-frequency speech sounds is a significant weakness of all passive BCDs, surgical or nonsurgical, this represents a significant advancement.

In the United States, active transcutaneous implants are not approved by the US Food and Drug Administration (FDA) for use in children younger than 12 years. This is in contrast to other parts of the world these devices are implanted in children as young as 5 years.[1,43] Therefore, current FDA-approved indications limit access to this technology for school-aged children.

MRI considerations. MRI compatibility needs to be taken into consideration for any child known to require postsurgical MRI. Percutaneous BCD implants are MRI safe with the external processor removed, although artifact will be generated if the brain is imaged. Some implants relying on magnetic coupling, both passive and active, have conditional FDA approval for MRI (see **Table 1**) with or without the magnet. Without FDA conditional approval for MRI with the magnet in situ, removal of the internal magnet (if removable) or device (if magnet not removable) is recommended.[48] Another consideration for choice of BCD implant is what area of the body requires imaging. A device with MRI approval without requiring magnet removal may be advantageous for children requiring body MRIs, because this would avoid surgical magnet removal and replacement. Artifact caused by the implant and magnet are not a concern for body imaging. However, the diagnostic utility of brain MRI will be impacted by the presence of a BCD implant. Selection of a device with a removable versus nonremovable magnet and surgical placement of the device in relationship to the brain area requiring imaging are important considerations when brain surveillance is required postimplantation. BCDs also cause artifact that will limit imaging of the brain by computer tomography.

HEARING REHABILITATION THROUGH BONE CONDUCTION DEVICES

Understanding the complex nature of BC hearing in children versus adults, and in pathologic ears, is important when considering the benefits and limitations of BCDs in the rehabilitation of childhood HL. At a minimum, BCDs should increase access to sound, ensuring audibility of speech at comfortable intensity levels. For children with congenital and early acquired HL, consideration of how intervention (or lack of intervention) with a BCD contributes to auditory development is also of importance.

The vast majority of children who are candidates for BCDs have permanent unilateral CHL.[49] There is an abundance of evidence that delayed intervention for childhood HL increases the risk for speech and language, academic, and developmental delays[23] even in mild and unilateral HL.[50–52] In such cases, BCDs not only provide listeners with increased access to speech, but potentially with bilateral auditory input that may influence binaural hearing abilities.

Binaural Hearing

The advantages binaural hearing provides are particularly important for children because much of their time will be spent in classrooms where significant background noise is typically present. Listening in adverse listening environments is enhanced by binaural hearing, which improves hearing in noise and provides directional hearing. In addition, there is some evidence that CHL negatively influences auditory cortex development and may result in central processing deficits.[53–56] The influence of unilateral and bilateral CHL on binaural hearing remains somewhat elusive. The cochleae of children with CHL have normal function and will be stimulated by the child's own vo-calizations and loud external sounds, likely contributing to development of binaural hearing pathways. Yet, research demonstrates that even children with unilateral CHL are at increased risk for speech, language, and academic delays.[57,58]

Individuals with unilateral CHL have difficulty understanding speech in noisy envi-ronments and decreased ability to locate sounds in the environment.[59] Studies have demonstrated that localization significantly improves using BCDs, although the spatial hearing provided by BCDs may not be equivalent to that achieved by those with normal hearing.[59–62] Limitations in providing early and consistent access to bilateral stimulation with BCDs during the critical auditory development years (ie, <5 years of age) may contribute to these gaps in performance. Studies in adults show that a nor-mally developed binaural hearing system can effectively extract binaural hearing cues through BCDs. Moreover, animal studies reveal that processing deficits arising from CHL can be reversed with time, supporting the notion that earlier and consistent inter-vention in children with CHL can promote binaural hearing and improved outcomes.[59,63]

Bilateral Bone Conduction Devices

In the case of bilateral hearing impairment, such as bilateral aural atresia, best out-comes are achieved with bilateral BCDs. Although bilateral fitting over each mastoid is not practical in infants who are unable to sit upright (see section on nonsurgical BCDs), children with bilateral CHL should be transitioned to bilateral fitting as early as possible. Bilateral BCD fitting maximizes access to sound and promotes auditory development. There is a wealth of evidence demonstrating that localization abilities, hearing in noise, audibility, and quality of life are improved in the bilateral BCD over unilateral BCD listening condition.[2,6,59,61,64–66] In addition, unilateral BCD fitting has been shown to have a negative impact on auditory ability by distorting timing cues.[37,62] Early bilateral stimulation with BCDs may promote development of binaural hearing.[62] Indeed, the healthy status of the cochleae in children with CHL may offer a prime opportunity to provide early stimulation to binaural pathways with BCDs during critical development years.

Bone Conduction Devices in Unilateral Hearing Loss

It is increasingly recognized that children with unilateral HL are at significantly greater risk than normal-hearing children for speech and language delays, reduced academic performance, and social emotional problems,[57,58,67] and the magnitude of these prob-lems in those with CHL seems to be less severe.[57,58,68] The consequences of unilateral HL can be difficult to identify, subtle, and delayed in presentation.[23,52] It is also possible that children with microtia are identified and offered other forms of early inter-vention that can mitigate the effects of unilateral HL.[57,68] Several researchers have pointed to the challenges in identifying the consequences of mild and/or unilateral HL, supporting a more conservative and preventative approach.[69]

It is known that increased access to words promotes better language development and better prepares children to enter school.[70] Children with unilateral HL, regardless of the cause, have reduced access to speech. In addition, they also have reduced or limited access to high-frequency sounds that are critical for speech and language development and require an increased signal-to-noise ratio to understand speech.[23]

The impairment or delay in speech and language caused by CHL in some children can go unrecognized until school age or overlooked entirely.[1,23,57] At present there is emerging evidence that delay in management can be consequential even if HL is conductive in nature. Kesser and colleagues[58] reported that 65% of school-aged children with unilateral aural atresia required some intervention or educational re-sources. Yet intervention is often delayed in these children.[2,5,57,69] In addition, cosmetic management of children with microtia/atresia has taken precedence over HL in some cases.[71] Given that early intervention has been shown to improve device compliance and speech and language outcomes, providers should counsel families regarding a balance between cosmetic concerns and other important benefits of BCD use.[4,57,71] Timely implementation of BCDs to address unilateral CHL in children with aural atresia should be a priority considering growing evidence that when these children are provided with BCDs as part of early intervention, their language and liter-acy are similar to normal-hearing peers.[68]

Severe to profound unilateral hearing loss

In addition to conductive or mixed loss, in cases of severe to profound unilateral sensorineural HL, often referred to as single sided deafness (SSD), a BCD can be used to reroute the signal similar to a contralateral routing of signal (CROS) hearing aid.[72] Studies of CROS aids have demonstrated improved speech recognition and reduced listening effort in dynamic classroom environments.[73,74] The literature on specific use of BCD for childhood SSD is sparse. However, neither CROS nor BCD re-stores binaural hearing or promotes binaural hearing development.[2,72,75]

A CROS aid is not an option until a fully open nonoccluding fitting of the ear canal can be achieved in the better hearing ear, which is not often achievable before age 6 to 7 years. In contrast, BCD may be used at a much younger age to increase access to speech and incidental learning. However, at this time, this approach to manage-ment of SSD is neither common nor considered best practice because longitudinal studies of benefit are lacking.

CLINICS CARE POINTS

- BCDs are a well-established and effective treatment solution for children with CHL who cannot be fitted with a traditional hearing aid. The most common indication in childhood is aural atresia.

- Infants with bilateral aural atresia should be fitted with a unilateral processor positioned along the forehead. These infants should be transitioned to a bilateral fitting over the mastoid as soon as permitted by the child's motor development.

- Children with unilateral aural atresia should be fitted early in life with a nonsurgical BCD as part of early intervention. The fitting should be transitioned to over the mastoid as soon as permitted by motor development.

- Direct drive active BCD implants provide better hearing and are associated with fewer skin problems than passive transcutaneous implant systems. These implants provide hearing equivalent to percutaneous implant systems that are best avoided in children. The drawback of active implant devices is that they are currently not FDA approved until age 12 years.

- The presence of a BCD implant may require surgical magnet or device removal before MRI. The presence of a BCD implant may also limit diagnostic utility of brain imaging.

REFERENCES

1. American Academy of Pediatrics JCoIH. Year 2007 position statement: principles and guidelines for early hearing detection and intervention programs. Pediatrics 2007;120(4):898–921.

2. Banga R, Doshi J, Child A, et al. Bone-anchored hearing devices in children with unilateral conductive hearing loss: a patient-carer perspective. Ann Otol Rhinol Laryngol 2013;122(9):582–7.

3. Fuchsmann C, Tringali S, Disant F, et al. Hearing rehabilitation in congenital aural atresia using the bone-anchored hearing aid: audiological and satisfaction results. Acta Otolaryngol 2010;130(12):1343–51.

4. Lloyd S, Almeyda J, Sirimanna KS, et al. Updated surgical experience with bone-anchored hearing aids in children. J Laryngol Otol 2007;121(9):826–31.

5. Ramakrishnan Y, Marley S, Leese D, et al. Bone-anchored hearing aids in children and young adults: the Freeman Hospital experience. J Laryngol Otol 2011;125(2):153–7.

6. Janssen RM, Hong P, Chadha NK. Bilateral bone-anchored hearing aids for bilateral permanent conductive hearing loss: a systematic review. Otolaryngol Head Neck Surg 2012;147(3):412–22.

7. Tjellstrom A, Hakansson B, Lindstrom J, et al. Analysis of the mechanical impedance of bone-anchored hearing aids. Acta Otolaryngol 1980;89(1–2):85–92.

8. Tonndorf J. Bone conduction. Studies in experimental animals. Acta Otolaryngol 1966;(Suppl 213):211+.

9. Stenfelt S. Bilateral fitting of BAHAs and BAHA fitted in unilateral deaf persons: acoustical aspects. Int J Audiol 2005;44(3):178–89.

10. Sohmer H, Freeman S. Further evidence for a fluid pathway during bone conduction auditory stimulation. Hearing Res 2004;193(1–2):105–10.

11. Khanna SM, Tonndorf J, Queller JE. Mechanical parameters of hearing by bone conduction. J Acoust Soc Am 1976;60(1):139–54.

12. Stenfelt S, Hakansson B. Air versus bone conduction: an equal loudness investigation. Hear Res 2002;167(1–2):1–12.

13. Nolan M, Lyon DJ. Transcranial attenuation in bone conduction audiometry. J Laryngol Otol 1981;95(6):597–608.

14. Vanniasegaram I, Bradley J, Bellman S. Clinical applications of transcranial bone conduction attenuation in children. J Laryngol Otol 1994;108(10):834–6.

15. Eeg-Olofsson M, Stenfelt S, Granstrom G. Implications for contralateral bone-conducted transmission as measured by cochlear vibrations. Otol Neurotol 2011;32(2):192–8.

16. Hulecki LR, Small SA. Behavioral bone-conduction thresholds for infants with normal hearing. J Am Acad Audiol 2011;22(2):81–92.

17. Small SA, Stapells DR. Maturation of bone conduction multiple auditory steady-state responses. Int J Audiol 2008;47(8):476–88.

18. Sohmer H, Freeman S, Geal-Dor M, et al. Bone conduction experiments in humans - a fluid pathway from bone to ear. Hear Res 2000;146(1–2):81–8.

19. Favoreel A, Heuninck E, Mansbach AL. Audiological benefit and subjective satisfaction of children with the ADHEAR audio processor and adhesive adapter. Int J Pediatr Otorhinolaryngol 2020;129:109729.

20. Verstraeten N, Zarowski AJ, Somers T, et al. Comparison of the audiologic results obtained with the bone-anchored hearing aid attached to the headband, the testband, and to the "snap" abutment. Otol Neurotol 2009;30(1):70–5.

21. Hakansson B, Tjellstrom A, Rosenhall U. Acceleration levels at hearing threshold with direct bone conduction versus conventional bone conduction. Acta Otolaryngol 1985;100(3–4):240–52.

22. Mylanus EA, Snik AF, Cremers CW. Influence of the thickness of the skin and subcutaneous tissue covering the mastoid on bone-conduction thresholds obtained transcutaneously versus percutaneously. Scand Audiol 1994;23(3):201–3.

23. Stelmachowicz PG, Pittman AL, Hoover BM, et al. The importance of high-frequency audibility in the speech and language development of children with hearing loss. Arch Otolaryngol Head Neck Surg 2004;130(5):556–62.

24. Pittman AL. Bone conduction amplification in children: stimulation via a percutaneous abutment versus a transcutaneous softband. Ear Hear 2019;40(6):1307–15.

25. van Barneveld D, Kok HJW, Noten JFP, et al. Determining fitting ranges of various bone conduction hearing aids. Clin Otolaryngol 2018;43(1):68–75.

26. Snik AF, Mylanus EA, Proops DW, et al. Consensus statements on the BAHA system: where do we stand at present? Ann Otol Rhinol Laryngol Suppl 2005;195:2–12.

27. Dun CA, Faber HT, de Wolf MJ, et al. Assessment of more than 1,000 implanted percutaneous bone conduction devices: skin reactions and implant survival. Otol Neurotol 2012;33(2):192–8.

28. Kraai T, Brown C, Neeff M, et al. Complications of bone-anchored hearing aids in pediatric patients. Int J Pediatr Otorhinolaryngol 2011;75(6):749–53.

29. Kiringoda R, Lustig LR. A meta-analysis of the complications associated with osseointegrated hearing aids. Otol Neurotol 2013;34(5):790–4.

30. Granstrom G, Bergstrom K, Odersjo M, et al. Osseointegrated implants in children: experience from our first 100 patients. Otolaryngol Head Neck Surg 2001;125(1):85–92.

31. Simms DL, Neely JG. Growth of the lateral surface of the temporal bone in children. Laryngoscope 1989;99(8 Pt 1):795–9.

32. Marsella P, Scorpecci A, D'Eredita R, et al. Stability of osseointegrated bone conduction systems in children: a pilot study. Otol Neurotol 2012;33(5):797–803.

33. Zeitoun H, De R, Thompson SD, et al. Osseointegrated implants in the management of childhood ear abnormalities: with particular emphasis on complications. J Laryngol Otol 2002;116(2):87–91.

34. Marsella P, Scorpecci A, Pacifico C, et al. Bone-anchored hearing aid (Baha) in patients with Treacher Collins syndrome: tips and pitfalls. Int J Pediatr Otorhinolaryngol 2011;75(10):1308–12.

35. Iseri M, Orhan KS, Kara A, et al. A new transcutaneous bone anchored hearing device - the Baha(R) attract system: the first experience in Turkey. Kulak Burun Bogaz Ihtis Derg 2014;24(2):59–64.

36. Reinfeldt S, Hakansson B, Taghavi H, et al. New developments in bone-conduction hearing implants: a review. Med Devices (Auckl) 2015;8:79–93.

37. Snapp H, Vogt K, Agterberg MJH. Bilateral bone conduction stimulation provides reliable binaural cues for localization. Hear Res 2020;388:107881.

38. Claros P, Diouf MS, Claros A. [Setting up a "Bonebridge"]. Rev Laryngol Otol Rhinol (Bord) 2012;133(4–5):217–20.

39. Zernotti ME, Di Gregorio MF, Galeazzi P, et al. Comparative outcomes of active and passive hearing devices by transcutaneous bone conduction. Acta Otolaryngol 2016;136(6):556–8.

40. Gawecki W, Gibasiewicz R, Marszal J, et al. The evaluation of a surgery and the short-term benefits of a new active bone conduction hearing implant - the Osia(R). Braz J Otorhinolaryngol 2020.

41. Gerdes T, Salcher RB, Schwab B, et al. Comparison of audiological results between a transcutaneous and a percutaneous bone conduction instrument in conductive hearing loss. Otol Neurotol 2016;37(6):685–91.

42. Ray J, Lau K, Moraleda J, et al. Soft-tissue outcomes following implantation of different types of bone conduction hearing devices in a single centre. J Laryngol Otol 2019;133(12):1079–82.

43. Sprinzl GM, Wolf-Magele A. The bonebridge bone conduction hearing implant: indication criteria, surgery and a systematic review of the literature. Clin Otolaryngol 2016;41(2):131–43.

44. Ellsperman SE, Nairn EM, Stucken EZ. Review of bone conduction hearing devices. Audiol Res 2021;11(2):207–19.

45. Mylanus EAM, Hua H, Wigren S, et al. Multicenter clinical investigation of a new active osseointegrated steady-state implant system. Otol Neurotol 2020;41(9): 1249–57.

46. Lau K, Scotta G, Wright K, et al. First United Kingdom experience of the novel Osia active transcutaneous piezoelectric bone conduction implant. Eur Arch Otorhinolaryngol 2020;277(11):2995–3002.

47. Goldstein MR, Bourn S, Jacob A. Early Osia(R) 2 bone conduction hearing implant experience: Nationwide controlled-market release data and single-center outcomes. Am J Otolaryngol 2021;42(1):102818.

48. Nospes S, Brockmann MA, Lassig A. [MRI in patients with auditory implants equipped with implanted magnets-an update: overview and procedural management]. Radiologe 2019;59(1):48–56.

49. Agterberg MBS, Breitholtz F, Christensen L, et al. Clinical guidance on bilateral fitting of bone conduction solutions in children and adults. Mölnlycke, Sweden: Cochlear Bone Anchored Solutions; 2018.

50. Bess FH, Dodd-Murphy J, Parker RA. Children with minimal sensorineural hearing loss: prevalence, educational performance, and functional status. Ear Hear 1998; 19(5):339–54.

51. Davis JM, Shepard NT, Stelmachowicz PG, et al. Characteristics of hearing-impaired children in the public schools: part II–psychoeducational data. J Speech Hear Disord 1981;46(2):130–7.

52. Bess FH, Tharpe AM. An introduction to unilateral sensorineural hearing loss in children. Ear Hear 1986;7(1):3–13.

53. Moore DR, Hine JE, Jiang ZD, et al. Conductive hearing loss produces a reversible binaural hearing impairment. J Neurosci 1999;19(19):8704–11.

54. Graydon K, Rance G, Dowell R, et al. Consequences of early conductive hearing loss on long-term binaural processing. Ear Hear 2017;38(5):621–7.

55. Xu H, Kotak VC, Sanes DH. Conductive hearing loss disrupts synaptic and spike adaptation in developing auditory cortex. J Neurosci 2007;27(35):9417–26.

56. Vasama JP, Makela JP, Parkkonen L, et al. Auditory cortical responses in humans with congenital unilateral conductive hearing loss. Hear Res 1994;78(1):91–7.

57. Jensen DR, Grames LM, Lieu JE. Effects of aural atresia on speech development and learning: retrospective analysis from a multidisciplinary craniofacial clinic. JAMA Otolaryngol Head Neck Surg 2013;139(8):797–802.

58. Kesser BW, Krook K, Gray LC. Impact of unilateral conductive hearing loss due to aural atresia on academic performance in children. Laryngoscope 2013;123(9): 2270–5.

59. Priwin C, Jonsson R, Hultcrantz M, et al. BAHA in children and adolescents with unilateral or bilateral conductive hearing loss: a study of outcome. Int J Pediatr Otorhinolaryngol 2007;71(1):135–45.

60. Agterberg MJ, Snik AF, Hol MK, et al. Contribution of monaural and binaural cues to sound localization in listeners with acquired unilateral conductive hearing loss:

improved directional hearing with a bone-conduction device. Hear Res 2012; 286(1–2):9–18.

61. Mylanus EA, van der Pouw KC, Snik AF, et al. Intraindividual comparison of the bone-anchored hearing aid and air-conduction hearing aids. Arch Otolaryngol Head Neck Surg 1998;124(3):271–6.

62. Priwin C, Stenfelt S, Granstrom G, et al. Bilateral bone-anchored hearing aids (BAHAs): an audiometric evaluation. Laryngoscope 2004;114(1):77–84.

63. Kaga K, Setou M, Nakamura M. Bone-conducted sound lateralization of interaural time difference and interaural intensity difference in children and a young adult with bilateral microtia and atresia of the ears. Acta Otolaryngol 2001;121(2): 274–7.

64. Dutt SN, McDermott AL, Burrell SP, et al. Patient satisfaction with bilateral bone-anchored hearing aids: the Birmingham experience. J Laryngol Otol Suppl 2002;(28):37–46.

65. Bosman AJ, Snik AF, van der Pouw CT, et al. Audiometric evaluation of bilaterally fitted bone-anchored hearing aids. Audiology 2001;40(3):158–67.

66. Dun CA, de Wolf MJ, Mylanus EA, et al. Bilateral bone-anchored hearing aid application in children: the Nijmegen experience from 1996 to 2008. Otol Neurotol 2010;31(4):615–23.

67. Lieu JE, Tye-Murray N, Fu Q. Longitudinal study of children with unilateral hearing loss. Laryngoscope 2012;122(9):2088–95.

68. Hyland A, Arnott WL, Rushbrooke E, et al. Outcomes for school-aged children with Aural Atresia. J Deaf Stud Deaf Educ 2020;25(4):411–20.

69. Brody R, Rosenfeld RM, Goldsmith AJ, et al. Parents cannot detect mild hearing loss in children. First place–Resident Clinical Science Award 1998. Otolaryngol Head Neck Surg 1999;121(6):681–6.

70. Hart B, Risley TR. Incidental teaching of language in the preschool. J Appl Behav Anal 1975;8(4):411–20.

71. Attaway J, Stone CL, Sendor C, et al. Effect of amplification on speech and language in children with Aural Atresia. Am J Audiol 2015;24(3):354–9.

72. Snapp HA, Hoffer ME, Liu X, et al. Effectiveness in rehabilitation of current wireless CROS technology in experienced bone-anchored implant users. Otol Neurotol 2017;38(10):1397–404.

73. Oosthuizen I, Picou EM, Pottas L, et al. Listening effort in school-aged children with limited useable hearing unilaterally: examining the effects of a personal, digital remote microphone system and a contralateral routing of signal system. Trends Hear 2021;25. 2331216520984700.

74. Picou EM, Davis H, Lewis D, et al. Contralateral routing of signal systems can improve speech recognition and comprehension in dynamic classrooms. J Speech Lang Hear Res 2020;63(7):2468–82.

75. Christensen L, Dornhoffer JL. Bone-anchored hearing aids for unilateral hearing loss in teenagers. Otol Neurotol 2008;29(8):1120–2.

Family-Centered and School-Based Enhancement of Listening and Spoken Language

Jenna Voss, PhD, CED, LSLS Cert AVEd

KEYWORDS

- Deaf/hard of hearing (DHH) • Family-centered • Auditory-based intervention
- Auditory verbal practice • Listening and spoken language • Interprofessional

KEY POINTS

- Children who are deaf/hard of hearing (DHH) can learn to listen and talk by using hearing technology, including cochlear implants and hearing aids, and auditory-based intervention.
- Interprofessional partnerships among otolaryngologists, audiologists, educators of the DHH, speech-language pathologists, general and special educators, and certified listening and spoken language specialists, are essential to family-centered care that supports children to listen and talk.
- Auditory verbal practice, a model of auditory-based intervention, emphasizes a family-centered, strengths-based approach to developmentally synchronous intervention.
- Children who are DHH benefit from various strategies and techniques from early intervention, through early childhood and into their school-aged classrooms as they navigate the development and advancement of auditory, receptive and expressive language, vocabulary, and pragmatic skills.
- Patient care networks and social services supports might be important for families with low access to services (ie, families without consistent insurance, families without access to in-person services or sufficient broadband for teleintervention, families without reliable transportation, and so forth).

INTRODUCTION AND BACKGROUND

Technological innovations, such as cochlear implants and hearing aids, provide access to sound for children who are deaf/hard of hearing (DHH). The result is parents choosing acquisition of listening and spoken language (LSL) as goals for their child, and children who are DHH effectively developing these skills. Communication modes of these children are varied, influenced by their family culture, communication opportunities and preferences, experiences, and values. Some children will use exclusively LSL; others will use a combination of sign and spoken language, and yet others will use primarily sign language for communication. Children who are DHH require

Fontbonne University, 6800 Wydown Boulevard, St. Louis, MO 63105, USA
E-mail address: jvoss@fontbonne.edu

Otolaryngol Clin N Am 54 (2021) 1219–1229
https://doi.org/10.1016/j.otc.2021.06.007
0030-6665/21/© 2021 Elsevier Inc. All rights reserved.

oto.theclinics.com

intervention and monitoring in a variety of areas: hearing technology, auditory and communication skill development, literacy and academic achievement, as well as social-emotional development.

An interprofessional team of physicians, audiologists, speech-language pathologists, and educators along with the child's caregivers and family members provides such intervention and monitoring. The child's otolaryngologist is an essential collaborator. The World Health Organization[1(p7)] defines interprofessional education and practice as, "two or more health professions learn about, from, and with each other to foster effective collaboration and improve the outcomes and quality of care." Through interprofessional practice, individuals are learning *about, from, and with* others—so they can serve children and families knowing the skills, strengths, and expertise that each person brings to the situation. With shared appreciation of the value of interprofessional practice, while equipped with institutional commitment to these collaborative models, team members can resist a preconceived hierarchy among professionals. Rather, each team member recognizes how collaboration and teamwork can best meet the child and family needs.

Children who are DHH might experience language delays in comparison to typically hearing peers owing to delays in diagnosis, fitting of hearing technology, and barriers to educational intervention. In addition, children might have additional disabilities that impact learning. Nevertheless, despite these challenges, many children who are DHH achieve necessary access to sound enabling them to use LSL as their primary mode of communication. When families of children who are DHH pursue hearing technology for their child to allow development of LSL skills, support from knowledgeable professionals is essential.

However, the knowledge and training of practitioners who support LSL intervention vary greatly, as the professional preparation programs for speech pathologists, audiologists, and educators of the deaf do not necessarily provide the clinical experience in working with children who are DHH learning LSL, but instead focus on supporting the development of signed languages. For this reason, families might need to prioritize professionals who provide auditory verbal practice.[2] Certified listening and spoken language specialists (LSLS cert auditory verbal educators and auditory verbal therapists) are professionals who have pursued advanced certification, including more than 900 hours of professional experience and 3 to 5 years of postgraduate mentoring, in auditory verbal practice.[3] These certified professionals include families as intervention and language partners, prioritize primacy of audition as the pathway for development of spoken language, maintain a focus on a developmental (rather than remedial) model of skill acquisition, and coach and guide caregivers (rather than didactic instruction), thus can be valuable members of the intervention team.

A STRONG START

The goals of the Early Hearing Detection and Intervention (EHDI) programs present in all 50 states are designed to achieve timely diagnosis and enrollment in early intervention programs. These programs typically follow recommendations set forth by the Joint Committee on Infant Hearing.[4] Current Joint Committee on Infant Hearing benchmarks are for the detection of hearing loss (by 1 month), diagnosis (by 3 months), and enrollment in intervention programs (by 6 months). Although medical homes, including audiologists and otologists, are primarily responsible for the provision of the hearing screening and diagnosis, a team of educators and therapists typically begins work with these children and families once the child is enrolled in an early intervention program. The parents' desired outcomes, their priorities and vision for their child's success, should guide the services and supports they will use during the early intervention and school-age years. By law, parents retain the power and authority to make intervention and educational decisions. The goal of early intervention is for families to receive coaching and instruction in varied topics related to hearing loss, device management, auditory and communication development, and facilitating development of home language, so that they develop the knowledge and skills to influence their child's learning trajectory positively.[5,6]

The timing of enrollment in early intervention, as well as the family's engagement and the experience of the LSL practitioner, determines the trajectory of the child's development and ultimately predicts academic achievement. Children receiving early intervention before 6 to 9 months of age achieve better outcomes than those enrolled later, across a range of communication skills.[7-10] Early intervention programs assist children in developing a strong foundation in language, literacy, and social and emotional domains, so it can be said that school readiness really begins at birth.[11] The success of the EHDI systems in the United States has resulted in many children entering the school system kindergarten-ready. However, children who are DHH, as a group, are at risk to have language lagging behind typically hearing children at school entry and may require more support for language development. Variability of school readiness is multifactorial and affected by length of unremedied hearing loss, quality and intensity of early intervention, and the child's cognition. Therefore, educators must provide ongoing monitoring and support for academic and social development of children who are DHH.

SUPPORTING SPOKEN LANGUAGE DEVELOPMENT THROUGH LISTENING

There is limited, but expanding, evidence-based research on the efficacy of specific strategies and techniques to promote LSL for children who are DHH.[12-14] However, a robust accumulation of evidence-informed practice guides LSL best practice.[15] Soman and Nevins[16] outline 5 core principles of LSL intervention. The principles provide a framework that can be individualized to deliver services in a culturally responsive manner:

1. Maximize learning to listen and learning through listening
2. Language and literacy development are foundational to all interventions
3. LSL is individualized, yet systematic, and richly multidimensional
4. Effective intervention is driven by interprofessional practice
5. Families are empowered to be partners in listening, spoken language, and literacy development

The practitioner's responsibility is to use these principles to educate parents in strategies and techniques to support LSL development. The goal is for the parents to become confident and competent in communicating with their child throughout daily routines in ways that maximize the child's listening, comprehension, and communication. Parents are coached to make simple changes, such as modifications to their child's listening environment, their response to child's communication, increasing wait time before responding to the child, or increasing their frequency of book sharing to impact LSL outcomes positively.[12,17]

AUDITORY ACCESS >> BRAIN DEVELOPMENT

Hearing is a first-order event in language development of children without hearing loss, as infants attend to the sounds in their environment and the voices of their caregivers. The infant brain rapidly develops the ability to discriminate the sounds of their native language.[18,19] The quantity and quality of linguistic input from parents impact typically hearing children's language development.[20-24]

For infants with hearing loss whose families' priority is spoken language, either exclusively or in combination with sign, consistent use of appropriately fit hearing technology can provide access to the sounds contained in spoken language. Amplification with hearing aids is particularly effective for hearing loss in the mild to moderate range. Children with greater degrees of loss can benefit from cochlear implant technology. Today's hearing technology provides the bottom-up acoustic signal needed by the brain.[25] This input is now available for top-down processing that encodes the acoustic signal enabling speech to be understood.[26,27] LSL intervention provides the brain training necessary for the DHH child to learn to optimize the more limited auditory input they receive.

Regardless of technology used and degree of hearing loss, children who are DHH are likely to have increased difficulty understanding the speech signal when background noise, including other talk, is present. Strategies to assist children who are DHH in classroom environments include preferential seating away from noise sources, use of Bluetooth streaming of the teacher's voice directly to their hearing device or devices, and physical modifications to the classroom, such as acoustic tile to reduce reverberation and excess noise. Collaboration between teachers and the child's personal and educational audiologist is essential to optimize access to sound. The otolaryngologist might be called on when medical treatment is needed to maintain consistent use of hearing technology, for example, when reversible middle ear dysfunction arises.

MODELS OF INTERVENTION: BIRTH TO 21 YEARS
Early Intervention

In the United States, the part C portion of the federal legislation, Individuals with Disabilities in Education Act (IDEA),[28] guides state-level implementation of early intervention programs for children from birth to age 3 years. The goal of early intervention is to mitigate developmental delay and to do so by educating the family as to how best help their child progress. Early intervention capitalizes on the concept of *developmental synchrony*,[29] where a child develops skills and abilities across domains at a synchronous rate, when their brain is most attuned to do so.

Families are assigned a service coordinator who oversees the development of an individual family service plan (IFSP) to ensure intervention services meet the child and family's needs. Eligibility criteria for services vary by state, as does the qualifications of the professionals providing services, and the frequency of services. In any early intervention context, practitioners are challenged to build on *family strengths* and attend to *family needs and priorities*,[30,31] while observing, modeling, reflecting, and jointly planning on the opportunities to enhance parent and child communication. There is a clear connection between the parent's language input and improved child language outcomes.[27,32] By identifying the *natural environments* where young children spend their time, intervention providers coach parents,[24,30] offering suggestions and models for making the most of these routine opportunities for communication.[31] When a parent is changing their child's diaper, an early intervention provider might offer *repetition* and *song*[12] as a strategy to increase auditory input and acoustically highlight important sounds or parts of speech. As a parent serves a toddler lunch, the early intervention provider might demonstrate the use of *wait time* and *expectant looks*[12,17] to prompt a child to make a verbal request for "more." While parents share a bedtime book with their child, the early intervention provider might challenge the family to engage in *labeling* and *naming* of pictures.[33,34]

In addition to support from professionals, in the early part of a family's journey, there is the need for *parent-to-parent* support.[35] Hands & Voices "Guide By Your Side" program[36] and the "Listen-Learn-Link-Parent-Support-Line" offered by the AG Bell Association[37] are 2 such models that connect families with others who have walked this path.

Early Childhood and School-Aged Intervention

The part B portion of the IDEA drives educational programming for children 3 to 21 years old. The focus of the law shifts to a child's ability to access the curriculum. Individualized Education Programs (IEPs) take the place of IFSPs to determine supports and services in the educational setting. This document is created by a team, including the parents and professionals, to identify the child's goals and related services and supports. During the school-age years, collaborative teams identify opportunities to target auditory, speech, and language practice within content instruction as a means to efficiently support overall development.[38–40] With intentional interprofessional practice, educators, speech-language pathologists, and audiologists collaborate to ensure continued development of grade-appropriate academic skills along with language and communication skills. Despite this shift in focus from family capacity building to curricular access, parents remain key influencers of child development and ideally should be engaged in their school-aged child's educational programming through ongoing communication with teachers and therapists.

Services and supports can be authorized across a range of settings depending on the learner's needs, with a focus on providing necessary supports in the *least restrictive environment*,[39] or education alongside typically developing peers to the maximum extent possible. Children might participate in specialized programs for children who are DHH or participate in general education settings alongside their typically developing peers. For some children, their IEP goals are addressed by an *itinerant teacher of the deaf*[39,41,42] or speech-language pathologist who visits their general education classroom for instruction. Periodic assessments in various domains provide ongoing monitoring of progress and ensure that appropriate services are being delivered. Results of these assessments inform eligibility for special education services. When benchmarks are not being met, intervention providers can shift strategies, intensity, or frequency of service delivery, instructional setting, or add services and supports.

Children who are DHH may use *accommodations*,[39] protected under the Americans with Disabilities Act, or *modifications*[39] to the curriculum, as authorized by the IEP, to ensure their access. Examples of commonly used accommodations for children who are DHH include communication access real-time translation reporting, dedicated note-takers, captioning, preferential seating, tutoring, extended testing time, and interpreters.

For some children, their hearing status might be a primary aspect of their identity, whereas others view it as but 1 aspect. In any case, attention to peer relationships, self-advocacy skills, and leadership skill development remains critically important to ensure the health and wellness of children who are DHH. Social groups, camps,[43] and activities specifically designed for children who are DHH provide important opportunities for adolescent and young adults to explore their unique identity, enhance self-confidence, including understanding of their strengths and abilities, and build pragmatic and advocacy skills in scaffolded, supportive environments. Private programs that focus on LSL development are a rich resource for this type of networking or to provide consultation and collaboration with public school programs that might have less experience supporting children who are DHH who use LSL.

SPECIAL CONSIDERATIONS FOR USE OF HEARING TECHNOLOGY AND INTERVENTION

Families with low access to services or supports need special considerations around use of hearing technology and intervention. Low access can be understood as range of limiting factors that influence successful outcomes with hearing technology, including inconsistent or limited insurance coverage and access to LSL intervention, unreliable transportation to and from appointments, and limited social supports. If the cochlear implant eligibility or care management team believes a family is at risk for low access to services, they can consider extending supports for the family beyond the initial period of postsurgical follow-up while also coordinating with social workers and the child's LSL service providers. These services might include the following:

- Help with scheduling appointments and education on the purpose of the appointments
- Additional support to access hearing technology and intervention services, including tele-medicine
- Arranging transportation
- Assistance for accessing insurance and other benefits
- Interpreting services
- Teleintervention or telemedicine options for LSL in areas where there is low access to these specialized providers
- Support with broadband access to receive teleservices
- Collaboration with other medical, therapeutic, or social service providers
- Ongoing support for retention of treatment (ie, tracking continuous use of the hearing technology through "wear time" data).

CLINICAL CARE/PATIENT CARE NETWORKS

COVID-19 has catapulted telemedicine and teleintervention services from what was a theoretic idea to an urgent reality in many locations. Many programs that provided in-person LSL services were required to pivot and begin providing services virtually. This created an opportunity for families who live in areas where there is low access to LSL-certified providers, such as rural communities, to connect virtually. A promising practice around telemedicine is a reduction of the number of visits needed to complete an eligibility/intake process into 1 visit with a specialist combined with telemedicine to complete the remaining appointments. For example, a family might receive the hearing aid eligibility and referral from an otologist via telemedicine, just before the initial hearing aid consultation appointment with the audiologist at the care center. Another example is relying on qualified LSL practitioners to troubleshoot challenges with hearing technology via telemedicine, instead of scheduling an in-center audiology appointment.

As systems recognize the benefit to families and overall efficiency in the expanded use of telemedicine and teleintervention, the creation of *clinical care networks* or *patient care networks* can address some challenges faced by families with low access. A medical or audiology center might audit all the steps in their eligibility and treatment process and identify opportunities for novel collaboration and coordination. The center could then establish patient-sharing agreements with several practitioners that are geographically dispersed across the state to provide services closer to the family's home. In addition, a treatment team could include an LSL practitioner as a standard member of the team to support those patients who used auditory-based intervention. The results of these patient care networks are that families are afforded more flexibility during the treatment process. In all of the scenarios and opportunities for reduced visits and expanded care networks, insurance billing and reimbursement can remain as significant barriers. If certain therapeutic services are not billable in a state (eg, auditory-based intervention provided by educators) or there are limits to cotreatment and telemedicine reimbursement, special permission or coordinated referrals might be necessary to prevent unanticipated charges or disjointed services.

GREAT EXPECTATIONS AND ENVIABLE OUTCOMES

Auditory-based LSL intervention can be used with children who are DHH from a range of lived experience and sociocultural backgrounds. It can support skill development for a range of children, including those who also use signed languages or alternative and augmentative communication. Early fitting of hearing technology coupled with family-centered intervention emphasizing auditory learning increases the number of children who are DHH who acquire spoken language contributing to stronger academic performance, improved social skills, and increased employment opportunities.[44] When families are engaged consistently as drivers of the intervention and professionals deliver services that assess and prioritize family needs, children who are DHH are best served. By maintaining high expectations[2] for all of the children and families served, professionals support families so their children can realize enviable lives.[45]

CLINICS CARE POINTS

- When not attended to, hearing loss can have a negative impact on spoken language acquisition, communication interactions, and ultimately, social and emotional development. This cascade of impact reaches educational outcomes, employment, and quality of life. However, with early diagnosis and the provision of intervention, one's risk for language delay is reduced and potential is realized.
- Engagement of the family in early intervention and school-based services is associated with better child language outcomes. Physicians can encourage family engagement and follow-through in their child's educational intervention by directly addressing this in medical visits and while counseling about hearing technology.
- When parents desire their child, who is deaf/hard of hearing, to learn to listen and talk, they will need consistent use of hearing technology and support from qualified professionals. Certified listening and spoken language specialist providers have specialized knowledge and skills to support the parents' confidence and competence in promoting listening and spoken language. To ensure children who are deaf/hard of hearing can maximize their use of hearing technology, they should be referred to and connected with families to systems of support.
- Assessment across domains of development, including audition, receptive and expressive language, and social skills, will ensure children who are deaf/hard of hearing are making sufficient progress and will identify when changes to intervention is warranted.

RESOURCES TO EXTEND LEARNING

Preparing to Teach, Committing to Learn: An Introduction to Educating Children Who Are Deaf/Hard of Hearing (2017-2020): this open-source e-book provides a strong overview of topics relative to deaf education in general, and auditory-based intervention for children learning listening and spoken language in particular. https://www.infanthearing.org/ebook-educating-children-dhh/index.html.

Videos of Auditory-Based Intervention, Cochlear Corporation: This site contains 10 full, unedited sessions provided by Certified Listening and Spoken Language Specialists, along with varied documentation including pre–cochlear implant and post–cochlear implant audiograms, session plans and associated goals. https://www.cochlear.com/intl/home/support/rehabilitation-resources/professional-resources/10-observation-lessons.

Strategies and Techniques: The following resources highlight varied strategies and techniques to use in auditory-based intervention.

> *Auditory Verbal Strategies to Build Listening and Spoken Language Skills*, by Fickenscher & Gaffney (2016). https://www.auditory-verbal-mentoring.com/downloads/downloads.php
>
> *Small Talk: Bringing Listening and Spoken Language to Your Young Child with Hearing Loss*, by Voss & White (2015). https://professionals.cid.edu/product/small-talk-bringing-listening-and-spoken-language-to-your-young-child-with-hearing-loss/
>
> Auditory Verbal Therapy. https://auditoryverbaltherapy.net/
>
> Listening Together. https://www.listeningtogether.com/

AG Bell Association: this nonprofit works toward a global mission of ensuring people who are deaf and hard of hearing have opportunities to listen and talk. https://www.agbell.org/

AG Bell Academy for Listening and Spoken Language: works to advance opportunities for children who are DHH to listen and talk through standards of excellence and certification of professionals who serve them. https://agbellacademy.org/

Hearing First https://www.hearingfirst.org/ & *Starts Hear Campaign* https://www.startshear.org

OPTIONSchools, Inc: a coalition of schools and affiliate members committed to ensure children with hearing loss and their families have access to listening and spoken language education choices. https://optionlsl.org/

Interprofessional Practice and Education, American Speech and Hearing Association (ASHA): https://www.asha.org/practice/interprofessional-education-practice/

ACKNOWLEDGMENTS

I thank my colleagues, Jessica Bergeroon and Uma Soman, for their assistance and expertise in preparation of this manuscript..

REFERENCES

1. Gilbert JH, Yan J, Hoffman SJ. A WHO report: framework for action on interprofessional education and collaborative practice. J Allied Health 2010;39(3):196–7.

2. Rosenzweig EA. Auditory verbal therapy: a family-centered listening and spoken language intervention for children with hearing loss and their families. Perspectives of the ASHA Special Interest Groups 2017;2(9):54–65.

3. About the Certification | The AG Bell Academy for listening and spoken language. Available at: https://www.agbell.org/AcademyDocument.aspx?id=541. Accessed March 1, 2017.

4. Joint Committee on Infant Hearing. Year 2019 position statement: principles and guidelines for early hearing detection and intervention programs. J Early Hear Detect Interv 2019;4(2):1–44.

5. Moeller MP, Carr G, Seaver L, et al. Best practices in family-centered early intervention for children who are deaf or hard of hearing: an international consensus statement. J Deaf Stud Deaf Educ 2013;18(4):429–45.

6. King A, Xu Y. Caregiver coaching for language facilitation in early intervention for children with hearing loss. Early Child Dev Care 2019;1–19.

7. Caselli N, Pyers J, Lieberman AM. Deaf children of hearing parents have age-level vocabulary growth when exposed to American Sign Language by 6 months of age. J Pediatr 2021;232:229–36.

8. Moeller MP. Early intervention and language development in children who are deaf and hard of hearing. Pediatrics 2000;106(3):e43.

9. Yoshinaga-Itano C. From screening to early identification and intervention: discovering predictors to successful outcomes for children with significant hearing loss. J Deaf Stud Deaf Educ 2003;8(1):11–30.

10. Ambrose SE, Walker EA, Unflat-Berry LM, et al. Quantity and quality of caregivers' linguistic input to 18-month and 3-year-old children who are hard of hearing. Ear Hear 2015;36(0 1):48S.

11. Meinzen-Derr J, Wiley S, Grove W, et al. Kindergarten readiness in children who are deaf or hard of hearing who received early intervention. Pediatrics 2020; 146(4):e20200557.

12. Fickenscher S, Salvucci D. Listening & spoken language strategies. In: Lenihan S, editor. Preparing to teach, committing to learn: an introduction to educating children who are deaf/hard of hearing. Utah: National Center for Hearing Assessment and Management; 2017.

13. Roberts MY, Curtis PR, Sone BJ, et al. Association of parent training with child language development: a systematic review and meta-analysis. JAMA Pediatr 2019. https://doi.org/10.1001/jamapediatrics.2019.1197.

14. Rosenzweig EA, Smolen ER. Providers' rates of auditory-verbal strategy utilization. Volta Rev 2021;120(2):79–95.

15. Eriks-Brophy A, Ganek H, DuBois G. Evaluating the research and examining outcomes of auditory-verbal therapy. In: Audit-verbal ther young child hear loss their fam pract who guide them. Plural Publishing; 2016. p. 35.

16. Soman U, Nevins ME. Guiding principles and essential practices of listening and spoken language intervention in the school-age years. Top Lang Disord 2018; 38(3):202–24.

17. MacIver-Lux K, Smolen ER, Rosenzweig EA, et al. Strategies for developing listening, talking, and thinking in auditory-verbal therapy. In: Auditory-verbal Therapy: science, research, and practice. Plural Publishing, Inc; 2020. p. 521–61.

18. Werker JF. Perceptual beginnings to language acquisition. Appl Psycholinguist 2018;39(4):703–28.

19. Maurer D, Werker JF. Perceptual narrowing during infancy: a comparison of language and faces. Dev Psychobiol 2014;56(2):154–78.

20. Hart B, Risley T. Meaningful differences in the everyday experience of young American children. Baltimore (MD): P.H. Brookes; 1995.

21. Romeo RR, Leonard JA, Robinson ST, et al. Beyond the 30-Million-Word Gap: Children's Conversational Exposure Is Associated With Language-Related Brain Function. Psychological Science 2018;29(5):700–10. https://doi.org/10.1177/0956797617742725.

22. Gilkerson J, Richards JA, Warren SF, et al. Language experience in the second year of life and language outcomes in late childhood. Pediatrics 2018;142(4): e20200557.

23. Anderson NJ, Graham SA, Prime H, et al. Linking Quality and Quantity of Parental Linguistic Input to Child Language Skills: A Meta-Analysis. Child Development 2021;92(2):484–501.

24. Sone BJ, Lee J, Roberts MY. Comparing Instructional Approaches in Caregiver-Implemented Intervention: An Interdisciplinary Systematic Review and Meta-Analysis. Journal of Early Intervention. February 2021. https://doi.org/10.1177/1053815121989807.

25. Kral A, Dorman MF, Wilson BS. Neuronal development of hearing and language: cochlear implants and critical periods. Annu Rev Neurosci 2019;42(1):47–65.

26. Kral A, Kronenberger WG, Pisoni DB, et al. Neurocognitive factors in sensory restoration of early deafness: a connectome model. Lancet Neurol 2016;15(6):610–21.

27. Niparko JK, Tobey EA, Thal DJ, et al. Spoken language development in children following cochlear implantation. JAMA J Am Med Assoc 2010;303(15):1498–506.

28. Part C of IDEA: early intervention for babies and toddlers. 2011. Available at: http://nichcy.org/laws/idea/partc. Accessed February 21, 2012.

29. Voss J, Stredler-Brown A. Getting off to a good start: practices in early intervention. In: Lenihan S, editor. Preparing to teach, committing to learn: an introduction to educating children who are deaf/hard of hearing. Utah; 2019. p. 8.1–8.18.

30. Rush D, Shelden M. The early childhood coaching handbook. 2nd edition. Baltimore (MD): Brookes Publishing; 2019.

31. McWilliam RA. Routines-based early intervention: supporting young children and their families. 1st edition. Baltimore (MD): Brookes Publishing; 2010.

32. Chu C, Dettman S, Choo D. Early intervention intensity and language outcomes for children using cochlear implants. Deaf Educ Int 2020;22(2):156–74.

33. DesJardin JL, Stika CJ, Eisenberg LS, et al. A longitudinal investigation of the home literacy environment and shared book reading in young children with hearing loss. Ear Hear 2017;38(4):441.

34. Dirks E, Wauters L. It takes two to read: interactive reading with young deaf and hard-of-hearing children. J Deaf Stud Deaf Educ 2018;23(3):261–70.

35. Henderson RJ, Johnson AM, Moodie ST. Revised conceptual framework of parent-to-parent support for parents of children who are deaf or hard of hearing: a modified Delphi study. Am J Audiol 2016;25(2):110–26.

36. Hands & voices. Guide by your Side™. 2020. Available at: http://www.handsandvoices.org/gbys/. Accessed February 27, 2021.

37. AG Bell Association for Deaf & Hard of Hearing. Listen-learn-link: parent support line. listen - learn - link parent support line. 2021. Available at: https://www.agbell.org/Families/Listen-Learn-Link-Parent-Support-Line. Accessed February 27, 2021.

38. White E. Listening and spoken language preschool programs. In: Lenihan S, editor. Preparing to teach, committing to learn: an introduction to educating children who are deaf/hard of hearing. Utah: National Center for Hearing Assessment and Management; 2017. Available at: http://www.infanthearing.org/ebook-educating-children-dhh/index.html. Accessed April 20, 2020.

39. Gettemeier D. Educational settings. In: Preparing to teach, committing to learn: an introduction to educating children who are deaf/hard of hearing. National Center for Hearing Assessment and Management; 2017. p. 10.1–10.14. Available at: https://www.infanthearing.org/ebook-educating-children-dhh/.

40. Soman UG, Kan D, Tharpe AM. Rehabilitation and educational considerations for children with cochlear implants. Otolaryngol Clin North Am 2012;45(1):141–53.

41. Luckner J. Providing itinerant services. In: *Deaf Learners: Developments in Curriculum and Instruction*. 1st Edition. Gallaudet University Press; 2006:93-111.
42. Luckner JL, Ayantoye C. Itinerant teachers of students who are deaf or hard of hearing: practices and preparation. J Deaf Stud Deaf Educ 2013;18(3):409–23.
43. AG Bell Association for Deaf & Hard of Hearing. LOFT: leadership opportunities for teens. LOFT. Available at: https://agbellloft.com. Accessed February 27, 2021.
44. Lim SR, Goldberg DM, Flexer C. Auditory-verbal graduates—25 years later: outcome survey of the clinical effectiveness of the listening and spoken language approach for young children with hearing loss. https://doi.org/10.17955/tvr.118.1.2.790.
45. Ann Turnbull: an enviable and dignified life. Available at: https://mn.gov/mnddc/ann-turnbull/ann-turnbull-02.html. Accessed February 26, 2021.

The Impact and Management of Listening-Related Fatigue in Children with Hearing Loss

Benjamin W.Y. Hornsby, PhD*, Hilary Davis, AuD, Fred H. Bess, PhD

KEYWORDS

- Pediatric hearing loss • Hearing loss • Fatigue • Listening-related fatigue
- Listening effort • Quality of life

KEY POINTS

- The listening difficulties of children with hearing loss (CHL) increase their susceptibility to severe listening-related fatigue and its significant, negative academic and psychosocial consequences.
- Professionals, including physicians, audiologists, and educators, should look for signs and symptoms of listening-related fatigue when working with CHL.
- Managing listening-related fatigue in CHL requires collaborative efforts of physicians, parents, the child, and other related professionals.
- Potential interventions can include educating the child, parents, and professionals working with the child about listening-related fatigue and its negative effects and implementation of active coping strategies to prevent or reduce its development.

INTRODUCTION

For most children, the act of listening and communicating successfully occurs naturally and effortlessly. However, for many children with hearing loss (CHL), this is not the case. The auditory information CHL receive might be degraded by their hearing loss, and/or distracting background noise, to such an extent that everyday listening situations can be challenging for them. Actively listening in such settings can require substantial mental effort for CHL.[1,2] This effortful listening, when sustained over time, can lead to feelings of fatigue. Subjective fatigue can be defined as a mood state associated with feelings of tiredness and exhaustion. Although many factors play a role in

Department of Hearing & Speech Sciences, Vanderbilt University School of Medicine, Vanderbilt Bill Wilkerson Center, Room 8310 Medical Center East, South Tower, 1215 21st Avenue South, Nashville, TN 37232-8242, USA
* Corresponding author.
E-mail address: ben.hornsby@vumc.org

Otolaryngol Clin N Am 54 (2021) 1231–1239
https://doi.org/10.1016/j.otc.2021.07.001
0030-6665/21/© 2021 Elsevier Inc. All rights reserved.

its development, evidence suggests fatigue is a direct consequence of sustained, high levels of mental or physical effort.[3] This is especially the case when the effort is applied toward a required task (eg, taking a test) rather than a personally desired goal (eg, playing a game). When the effort is applied toward listening tasks, the resultant fatigue is referred to as *listening-related fatigue*.[4–6]

If the feelings of fatigue are severe and recurrent, substantial negative consequences might be observed in children and adults. For example, cognitive processing skills, such as the ability to maintain focus and attention, are often degraded in a fatigued state.[3,7–10] Adding to these cognitive issues, severe, recurrent fatigue can disrupt sleep patterns leading to an increased need for sleep and rest during the day.[11] In addition, feelings of fatigue are associated with psychosocial issues, such as depression and emotional difficulties.[12–14] Clearly these diverse issues have the potential to impose negative aftereffects on children at home and at school. Research on the functional impact of fatigue on CHL is limited; however, work in children with other chronic health issues for which fatigue is a primary complaint (eg, cancer, cerebral palsy, chronic fatigue syndrome) can provide some insight. Research in these populations suggests that in the school setting, fatigued children are more likely to perform poorly academically, repeat a grade, and be absent from school. In addition, these children are more likely to disengage from their typical daily activities and experience disruptions in their social relationships.[15–20]

There is mounting evidence to support the hypothesis that CHL are at risk for experiencing significant fatigue.[6,21–24] For example, Hornsby and colleagues[22,23] used a generic subjective fatigue scale, the Pediatric Quality of Life-Multidimensional Fatigue Scale[25] (PedsQL-MFS), to quantify fatigue in children with mild to severe hearing loss and control groups of children without hearing loss. There was some variation across studies; however, the primary conclusion was that CHL experienced more fatigue than children without hearing loss. The investigators also compared the fatigue reported by CHL to that of children with other chronic health conditions. Results showed that the fatigue experienced by CHL was similar to, *or greater than*, that experienced by children with cancer, multiple sclerosis, rheumatoid arthritis, and other significant health conditions,[23] highlighting the potential impact of fatigue on CHL (**Fig. 1**).

Importantly, the impact of hearing loss on fatigue in adults and children does not appear to be dependent on the magnitude of their hearing loss. For example, Hornsby and Kipp[26] found no association between degree of hearing loss and fatigue, or vigor, ratings in a large sample of adults (N = 143). In that sample, hearing losses in the better-hearing ear (pure-tone-average [PTA] of thresholds at 500, 1000, and 2000 Hz) ranged from about 8 dB hearing loss to 95 dB hearing loss. Hornsby and colleagues[23] reported a similar finding based on results from a sample of CHL (N = 60) whose better-ear PTA ranged from 5 to 68 dB hearing loss. Likewise, evidence suggests that even having a unilateral hearing loss increases risk for fatigue in adults[27] with hearing loss and CHL.[24] Alhanbali and colleagues[27] examined fatigue ratings between 4 groups of adults (N = 50 per group) with the following: (1) unilateral hearing loss, (2) bilateral hearing loss and wearing hearing aids, (3) cochlear implant users, and (4) an age-matched control group without hearing loss. All groups with hearing loss reported significantly more fatigue than the control group. However, there were no differences in fatigue ratings across the hearing loss groups. Bess and colleagues[24] reported a similar finding when comparing fatigue ratings, obtained via parent-proxy report, between children without hearing loss and those with unilateral or bilateral hearing loss. These findings are important and highlight the increased risk for fatigue-related issues in children with even mild, or unilateral, hearing impairments.

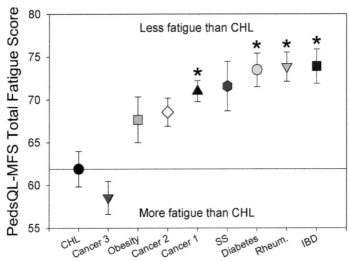

Fig. 1. Mean fatigue ratings of CHL (from Hornby and colleagues, 2017; *black filled circle, far left*) and children with other chronic health conditions, including 3 studies on cancer, 1 study on obesity, short stature (SS), diabetes, rheumatoid arthritis, and inflammatory bowel disease (IBD), respectively (see Hornsby and colleagues, 2017 for details). Fatigue ratings are the total score obtained using the PedsQL-MFS (Varni and colleagues, 2002). Note that lower scores on this measure denote increased fatigue. Error bars = 1 standard error. The solid black line represents the total fatigue score of the CHL from Hornsby and colleagues (2017). Groups with mean scores above, or below, the black line reported less or more total fatigue, respectively, than the CHL. * PedsQL-MFS total scores were from groups who reported significantly LESS fatigue than CHL (* groups have significantly higher PedsQL-MFS scores). Significance is based on Welch's *t* test for unequal variances with significance determined by Bonferroni correction. (*Data from* Hornsby BWY, Gustafson SJ, Lancaster H, et al. Subjective fatigue in children with hearing loss assessed using self-and parent-proxy report. Am J Audiol 2017;26(3S):393-407.

IDENTIFICATION AND MANAGEMENT OF LISTENING-RELATED FATIGUE IN CHILDREN WITH HEARING LOSS

Although CHL might be more likely to experience fatigue-related problems, clearly not all CHL will struggle with *severe* listening-related fatigue. Severe fatigue has functional academic or psychosocial consequences that are impactful enough to warrant monitoring or intervention. Development of severe fatigue is associated with many factors, in addition to the applied effort on a task.[3] For listening-related fatigue, Davis and colleagues[5] argue that task factors, such as listening difficulty, duration of listening, and any negative consequences for errors during listening, all play a role. Likewise, subject factors, such as the individual's motivation to understand, their applied listening effort, and their sense of control over the listening task (eg, can they implement a coping strategy to improve the listening situation) can influence whether significant fatigue develops in response to the listening challenges.[3,5]

Given the multitude of factors at play, it is not surprising that listening-related fatigue can be a problem for children regardless of their degree or type of hearing loss. Children suspected of fatigue should be given a subjective fatigue evaluation to confirm the presence of fatigue and to understand better the intensity and characteristics of the symptoms. Although currently, only generic scales (eg, PedsQL-MFS) are available, the authors' laboratory is developing a measure specific to listening-related fatigue: the Vanderbilt Fatigue Scales (VFS). The authors believe these scales will be useful for identifying those children with the most significant difficulties (see Bess and colleagues[24] for details). Once complete, the scales will be made available for general clinical, educational, and research use. In the interim, physicians, and other professionals who work with these children, should become familiar with the symptoms and behaviors that are commonly associated with listening-related fatigue. Davis and colleagues[6] explored listening-related fatigue in CHL by conducting focus groups and interviews with CHL (and their parents and the teachers/professionals that work with them) and asking them directly about fatigue-related issues they experience. The comments of CHL mirrored many made by adults with hearing loss[5] and confirmed that listening-related fatigue is a significant problem for some CHL. The experiences, behaviors, and feelings associated with listening-related fatigue in CHL are diverse, having physical, cognitive, and social-emotional effects. Per focus group discussions, common signs and symptoms include being off-task or "zoning out" during lectures, a perceived decrease in energy, and child complaints of being tired or weary. **Table 1** lists common flags for listening-related fatigue. This knowledge is important to ensure clinicians provide appropriate counseling to CHL, their families, and educators.

To date, no empirically validated interventions have been developed that specifically target listening-related fatigue in CHL. Until such interventions are developed, professionals should consider the following issues and approaches for management options for those children most affected by listening-related fatigue (**Table 2**). Physicians are encouraged to discuss listening-related fatigue and potential management strategies with their patients with hearing loss and their families. These recommendations and points for consideration are based on discussions concerning listening-related fatigue that were held during focus group/interviews with CHL, their parents, and school professionals.[6]

Table 1	
Red flags for severe listening-related fatigue in children with hearing loss	
Fatigue Domains	**Signs and Symptoms**
Physical	• Reports feeling tired, exhausted, drained, and/or worn out from listening • Develops headaches following sustained listening • Requires naps, additional sleep, and/or silent time to recover from listening-fatigue • Needs regular "listening" breaks at school to reduce development of listening-fatigue • Reports disrupted sleep patterns • Frequently removes their hearing devices to avoid, or recover from, listening-fatigue
Cognitive	• Has difficulty **maintaining effort and attention on a task** (eg, "zone out"), even routine mental tasks, following a period of sustained listening • With severe listening-related fatigue, the child may consciously disengage from mental activities (eg, **shuts down, gives up**)
Social-emotional	• Becomes extremely **sad, upset, angered, stressed, and/or emotionally exhausted** in response to listening difficulties, particularly in social settings • Reports that listening difficulties in social settings are fatiguing and may **avoid social settings** to cope with listening fatigue

Table 2
Managing listening-related fatigue in children with hearing loss

Important Considerations	Management Recommendations
Observe the child in their typical listening environment	• Review child's typical listening and learning environments, including the classroom, gymnasium, cafeteria, and during group interactions. • Observe the child in a variety of settings to determine if specific situations or locations are more fatiguing • Look for fatigue-related behaviors in these situations (see **Table 1**) • Discuss challenging listening situations with the CHL to understand their day-to-day experiences with fatigue
Optimize the listening environment	• Minimize background noise and reverberation with acoustical treatments (eg, curtains, carpeting) and turning off noisy equipment (eg, air conditioning units) when possible • Reduce visual distractions (eg, other students or cluttered spaces) • Use good communication skills when speaking to a CHL. Ensure the child has access to the speaker's face and is close to them to reduce difficulties of listening at a distance
Ensure consistent use of amplification	• Verify the child's amplification (eg, hearing aids, cochlear implants, bone anchored devices, remote microphone systems) are fit according to prescriptive targets and are functioning appropriately • Consistent use of amplification should be the gold standard; however, sustained listening through a device can be fatiguing for some children and a break from device use may be needed (see accommodations point below)
Provide accommodations	• Allow CHL to use preferential, flexible seating for optimal visual and auditory access in the classroom setting • Provide "listening breaks"—times where the student is permitted to take a break from attentive listening in the classroom, particularly after a period of difficult listening. Examples include taking a short movement break like standing and stretching or going to the restroom or for a water break. Alternatively, the child may take a break from work while remaining at their desk and/or remove their assistive devices (eg, hearing aid, cochlear implants) for a short period of time
Consider the daily schedule	• Schedule potentially fatiguing, auditory-heavy tasks (eg, speech-language therapy) or classroom activities (eg, listening to lectures or group discussions) at a time when the child is less likely to become fatigued. Many teachers reported scheduling these in the morning resulted in less fatigue

LISTENING-RELATED FATIGUE IN CHILDREN WITH HEARING LOSS: COUNSELING AND EDUCATION

Interestingly, some children struggled to recognize their own difficulties with fatigue in challenging listening situations.[6] If children are unaware of their struggles, they might be less likely to know how to recover, or request support in these situations. Therefore, it is important for physicians, and other professionals, working with CHL to have an understanding of listening-related fatigue and its negative effects. This information can help guide counseling of CHL, and their families, about the possibility of fatigue-related difficulties.[21,24,28] For example, professionals might discuss with children how their hearing loss can impact them in challenging listening situations and introduce them to the construct of listening-related fatigue, and how it can be expressed in different ways (ie, physically, socially, emotionally, and cognitively). For CHL who are experiencing fatigue-related issues (see **Table 1**), it could also be helpful to discuss coping strategies the child can use to limit, or recover from, listening-related fatigue. Finally, it would be important for professionals working with these children to encourage and promote the child's self-advocacy skills. This can include teaching them how to voice their concerns with others (eg, other health care providers or educators) and how to request an intervention plan if they cannot implement a change in their own environment. Some CHL express a desire to use various coping strategies but do not feel they have enough control over their schedule or listening environment to do so.[6] For example, a child might experience a headache and/or fatigue after an extended period of active listening and might want to turn off their hearing devices for a few minutes to recover and recharge. If the teacher working with the child is unaware of their fatigue-related issues, they might not be supportive of the child removing their devices. As a professional working with the child, how could you help the child develop a plan to request this intervention? Educating the child and those who work with them about the potential effects that difficult listening, and subsequent listening-related fatigue, can cause is paramount for implementing effective interventions. Ongoing discussions regarding fatigue-related interventions, both in school and in the home, might be required to help some CHL succeed. **Table 3** provides a summary of these counseling and education key points.

Table 3 Counseling and education key points	
Child education	• Discuss challenging listening situations and fatigue-associated difficulties • Consider action plans for requesting interventions as needed to develop self-advocacy skills
Parent education	• Counsel parents about signs, and possible negative effects, of listening-related fatigue • Provide strategies and suggestions for at-home management if fatigue is experienced, such as rest breaks or amplification breaks
Professional education	• Educate other professionals about the signs of, and possible negative effects, of listening-related fatigue • Engage in multidisciplinary collaboration by using a team approach to determine appropriate intervention and management plans for each child

SUMMARY

There is mounting evidence to support the premise that CHL are at increased risk for listening-related fatigue and its associated sequelae. This article offers a brief overview of listening-related fatigue in CHL, including definitions of fatigue, its importance and possible consequences, and recommended considerations for the identification and management of fatigue in pediatric hearing loss. Although many fatigue scales have been developed for children with other medical conditions, no such instrument has been designed specifically for CHL. To meet this need, the authors are in the final stages of developing the VFS, a child-centered tool that can be used for the identification of listening-related fatigue in children with hearing impairment. Clearly, the need for additional research on listening-related fatigue is essential, as information is lacking related to prevalence, side effects, causes, and evidenced-based management strategies. Specific areas of needed research include examining listening-related fatigue as a function of age, degree, and type of hearing loss and to assess the responsiveness of the VFS to different intervention strategies. Finally, a need exists for developing evidence-based interventions designed to reduce fatigue in CHL; an obvious example is to explore whether different amplification devices play a role in the reduction of listening-related fatigue.

CLINICS CARE POINTS

- Ask the child with hearing loss, and/or their parents, about the issue of listening-related fatigue. Some children with hearing loss may report behaviors consistent with listening-related fatigue but may be unaware of its relationship to their hearing difficulties.

- The experience of listening-related fatigue can vary widely in children with hearing loss, having physical, cognitive, and social-emotional manifestations.

- Children with hearing loss may be at increased risk for fatigue-related problems regardless of whether their hearing loss is unilateral or bilateral, or whether the loss is mild or severe.

- Educate and advocate-- educate children with hearing loss, their parents, and other professionals that work with these children with hearing loss about listening-related fatigue and its negative sequelae. Encourage and teach children with hearing loss to be advocates for themselves and take active steps to manage listening-related fatigue in their lives.

- Providing brief listening breaks, with or without hearing devices, may provide some relief for children struggling with listening-related fatigue.

DISCLOSURE

This work was supported by the Institute of Education Sciences (IES), U.S. Department of Education, via a grant awarded to Vanderbilt University Medical Center (#R21DC012865; Bess, PI). The opinions expressed are those of the authors and do not represent the views of the Institute or the U.S. Department of Education.

REFERENCES

1. Hicks CB, Tharpe AM. Listening effort and fatigue in school-age children with and without hearing loss. J Speech Lang Hear Res 2002;45:573–84.
2. McGarrigle R, Gustafson S, Hornsby B, et al. Behavioral measures of listening effort in school-age children: examining the effects of signal-to-noise ratio, hearing loss, and amplification. Ear Hear 2019;40(2):381–92.

3. Hockey GR. A motivational control theory of cognitive fatigue. In: The psychology of fatigue: work, effort and control. New York, NY: Cambridge University Press; 2013. p. 132–54.

4. Pichora-Fuller M, Kramer S, Eckert M, et al. Hearing impairment and cognitive energy: the framework for understanding effortful listening (FUEL). Ear Hear 2016; 37(1):5S–27S.

5. Davis H, Schlundt D, Bonnet K, et al. Understanding listening-related fatigue: perspectives of adults with hearing loss. Int J Audiol 2020;60(6):458–68.

6. Davis H, Schlundt D, Bonnet K, et al. Listening-related fatigue in children with hearing loss: perspectives of children, parents, and school professionals. Am J Audiol 2021. in review.

7. Boksem M, Tops M. Mental fatigue: costs and benefits. Brain Res Rev 2008;59(1): 125–39.

8. Hopstaken J, van der Linden D, Bakker A, et al. A multifaceted investigation of the link between mental fatigue and task disengagement. Psychophysiology 2014;52(3):305–15.

9. Moore T, Key A, Thelen A, et al. Neural mechanisms of mental fatigue elicited by sustained auditory processing. Neuropsychologia 2017;106:371–82.

10. Gustafson S, Key A, Hornsby B, et al. Fatigue related to speech processing in children with hearing loss: behavioral, subjective, and electrophysiological measures. J Speech Lang Hear Res 2018;61(4):1000–11.

11. Roscoe J, Kaufman M, Matteson-Rusby S, et al. Cancer-related fatigue and sleep disorders. Oncologist 2007;12(S1):35–42.

12. Visser M, Smets E. Fatigue, depression and quality of life in cancer patients: how are they related? Support Care Cancer 1998;6(2):101–8.

13. Hockenberry-Eaton M, Hinds P, Howard V, et al. Developing a conceptual model for fatigue in children. Eur J Oncol Nurs 1999;3(1):5–11.

14. Grillon C, Quispe-Escudero D, Mathur A, et al. Mental fatigue impairs emotion regulation. Emotion 2015;15(3):383–9.

15. Stoff E, Bacon M, White P. The effects of fatigue, distractibility, and absenteeism on school achievement in children with rheumatic diseases. Arthritis Care Res 1989;2(2):49–53.

16. Berrin S, Malcarne V, Varni J, et al. Pain, fatigue, and school functioning in children with cerebral palsy: a path-analytic model. J Pediatr Psychol 2006;32(3): 330–7.

17. McCabe M. Fatigue in children with long-term conditions: an evolutionary concept analysis. J Adv Nurs 2009;65(8):1735–45.

18. Ravid S, Afek I, Suraiya S, et al. Kindergarten children's failure to qualify for first grade could result from sleep disturbances. J Child Neurol 2009;24(7):816–22.

19. Ravid S, Afek I, Suraiya S, et al. Sleep disturbances are associated with reduced school achievements in first-grade pupils. Dev Neuropsychol 2009;34(5):574–87.

20. Beebe D. Cognitive, behavioral, and functional consequences of inadequate sleep in children and adolescents. Pediatr Clin North Am 2011;58(3):649–65.

21. Bess F, Hornsby B. Commentary. Ear Hear 2014;35(6):592–9.

22. Hornsby B, Werfel K, Camarata S, et al. Subjective fatigue in children with hearing loss: some preliminary findings. Am J Audiol 2014;23(1):129–34.

23. Hornsby B, Gustafson S, Lancaster H, et al. Subjective fatigue in children with hearing loss assessed using self- and parent-proxy report. Am J Audiol 2017; 26(3S):393–407.

24. Bess F, Davis H, Camarata S, et al. Listening-related fatigue in children with unilateral hearing loss. Lang Speech Hear Serv Sch 2020;51(1):84–97.

25. Varni J, Burwinkle T, Katz E, et al. The PedsQL™ in pediatric cancer. Cancer 2002;94(7):2090–106.
26. Hornsby B, Kipp A. Subjective ratings of fatigue and vigor in adults with hearing loss are driven by perceived hearing difficulties not degree of hearing loss. Ear Hear 2016;37(1):e1–10.
27. Alhanbali S, Dawes P, Lloyd S, et al. Self-reported listening-related effort and fatigue in hearing-impaired adults. Ear Hearing 2017;38(1):e39–48.
28. Bess FH, Gustafson SJ, Hornsby BWY. How hard can it be to listen? Fatigue in school-age children with hearing loss. J Educ Audiol 2014;20:1–14.

Vestibular Evaluation and Management of Children with Sensorineural Hearing Loss

Melissa Hazen, MSc, AUD(C)[a,b,c],
Sharon L. Cushing, MD, MSc, FRCSC[a,b,c,d],*

KEYWORDS

- Vestibular dysfunction • Sensorineural hearing loss • Bilateral vestibular impairment
- Cochlear implants

KEY POINTS

- Vestibular impairment is common in children with sensorineural hearing loss
- Screening for vestibular and balance impairment in children is feasible
- Developmental consequences of vestibular impairment
  - Exist
  - Extend beyond balance
  - Impact outcome
- Cochlear implants impact vestibular function
- Abnormal vestibular function increases risk of cochlear implant device failure related to trauma
- Management options exist and are expanding

BACKGROUND

Vestibular Dysfunction is Common in Children with Sensorineural Hearing Loss

Sensorineural hearing loss (SNHL) is the most common congenital sensory impairment, occurring in 3 of every 1000 live births.[1] The prevalence of vestibular dysfunction (VD) in children with SNHL is significant, with estimates ranging between 20% and 70%.[2–6] Our own studies demonstrate that 35% of children with profound bilateral SNHL have severe or absent vestibular function. However, when more subtle dysfunction is included, 50% have evidence of end-organ vestibular abnormalities.[2,7] It is

[a] Department of Communication Disorders, Hospital for Sick Children, 555 University of Toronto, 6103C Burton Wing, Toronto, Ontario M5G1X8, Canada; [b] Archie's Cochlear Implant Laboratory, Hospital for Sick Children, Toronto; [c] Department of Otolaryngology, Head & Neck Surgery, University of Toronto; [d] Institute of Medical Sciences, University of Toronto
* Corresponding Author. Hospital for Sick Children, 555 University of Toronto, 6103C Burton Wing, Toronto, Ontario M5G1X8, Canada.
E-mail address: Sharon.cushing@sickkids.ca

Otolaryngol Clin N Am 54 (2021) 1241–1251
https://doi.org/10.1016/j.otc.2021.08.001
0030-6665/21/© 2021 Elsevier Inc. All rights reserved.

important to understand that most children with SNHL and VD (SNHL-VD) do not present with vertigo. Dysfunction of the vestibular end-organs in these children presents with motor milestone delays and balance impairments[8,9]; this is particularly true when VD is nonprogressive, severe, congenital and/or bilateral, which is often the case in children with significant bilateral SNHL.

There are motor, neurocognitive, behavioral, and functional implications of VD on a developing child.[8] Although an early diagnosis is beneficial with regard to counseling, intervention is necessary to improve balance in these children and promote their physical, spatial, and neurocognitive development.[3,6,8]

The relationship between auditory and vestibular function is variable, although patterns linked to the cause and degree of SNHL do exist.[10–13] Specifically, the risk of vestibular dysfunction co-occurring with balance dysfunction is highest in children with severe to profound SNHL. This condition is particularly true when the underlying cause is (1) an acquired infectious disease (ie, meningitis), congenital cytomegalovirus; (2) a syndromic cause (ie, Usher type 1 syndrome); or (3) cochleovestibular anomalies (ie, enlarged vestibular aqueduct).[14–27] In addition, VD is reported to occur in thalidomide fetopathy, kernicterus, nonsyndromic autosomal recessive-type SNHL, as well as SNHL of unknown cause.[10] The vestibular "phenotype" of many causes of SNHL remains to be defined.

Identifying the cause of SNHL may aid in estimating the likelihood of concurrent VD, and conversely, knowing that the child has SNHL-VD may guide the etiologic workup. Given the high prevalence of VD in association with SNHL and the absence of what many clinicians would consider typical clinical vestibular symptoms, children presenting with SNHL should be routinely screened for vestibular and balance dysfunction.[3,28–30]

DISCUSSION
Feasibility of Screening for Vestibular and Balance Impairment in Children

Despite the high probability of concomitant SNHL and VD, and the advantage of early identification of this VD, until recently only a small portion of children with SNHL underwent evaluation or screening of vestibular function. There is now greater appreciation of the benefits of identifying VD, and that screening, as well as more comprehensive evaluation, may be accomplished in children. For these reasons, screening for VD is increasing. This article focuses on a practical screening algorithm that can be applied in the busy clinical setting.

Screening balance and vestibular assessment includes at least one of the following, and ideally all 3 components:

1. Historical review of motor milestones
2. Direct assessment of balance
3. Direct assessment of horizontal canal function (applicable to infants younger than 6 months)

Review of motor milestones
Asking caregivers about neck control as an infant and age at sitting and walking independently can provide important insight into the coexistence of a VD. Timelines for each of these milestones are outlined in **Table 1**.

Assessment of balance
Often lack of age-appropriate balance skills is not obvious during routine office evaluation of children with SNHL. However, when children with SNHL-VD are challenged by difficult balance tasks relying upon the peripheral vestibular system, deficiencies in

Table 1 Red flags for motor milestones[94]	
Motor Milestone	**Timeframe**
Absence of head control	4 mo
Unable to sit unsupported	7–9 mo
Unable to crawl/bottom shuffle	12 mo
Not attempting to walk	18 mo

balance function will surface.[31,32] Our preferred clinical test is the balance subset of the Oseretsky Test of Motor Proficiency-2 (BOT-2). BOT-2 is our standard measure of balance in children older than 4 years.[33] The BOT-2 is a battery of 9 tasks for which reference normative data are available. The tasks are performed under different conditions (ie, eyes open or eyes closed), and some require use of a standardized balance beam. Therefore, use of the entire balance subtest of the BOT-2 in a busy clinical setting is not feasible.

To identify a useful screening assessment of balance in children, our research group evaluated the BOT-2 battery. Sensitivity, specificity, and practicality of each test were reviewed. The one-foot standing with eyes open and eyes closed was the most effective screening tool.[30] This tool does require specific equipment (ie, balance beam), takes several minutes to complete, and standardized normative data are readily available. Therefore, it is ideally suited for screening purposes. **Table 2** outlines the duration of expected one-foot standing by age.

Assessment of horizontal canal function

A head impulse test, also known as a head thrust maneuver or the Halmagyi maneuver, can be done to screen for horizontal canal function and will identify side-specific abnormalities of the vestibulo-ocular reflex (VOR). Specifically, this test is performed by having the child fixate on a stationary target and the head is rapidly (high frequency, low amplitude) rotated left or right. Children with abnormal horizontal canal function leading to a deficient VOR will not be able to maintain stationary gaze on the target, and the tester will appreciate corrective saccades back to the target. Use of a novel and interesting target allows this test to be completed in young children.

In addition to the head impulse test described earlier, infants younger than 6 months can also be assessed for postrotary nystagmus without the use of any specialized equipment to eliminate visual fixation (ie, Frenzel goggles) that would be required in older children and adults, because this test capitalizes on the inability of young infants to suppress the VOR response. This evaluation can be done in the office by spinning the child (and the caregiver on whose lap they sit) on a stool and immediately afterward examining for postrotary nystagmus. The key normal examination finding is postrotary nystagmus with the fast phase directed away from the direction of acceleration, which indicates an intact horizontal VOR.[34] Given the qualitative nature of this assessment (present or absent) it is useful in detecting bilateral and complete horizontal canal dysfunction; however, it may be more limited in identifying incomplete or unilateral dysfunction. Owing to the 6-month upper age limit, we often use this test in infants who have come in for hearing loss evaluation following a failed newborn hearing screening.

Ideally, all 3 components of the screening assessment are performed in young children with SNHL. However, completion of any single step can contribute to the identification of children likely to have VD.

Table 2
Expected and red flag one-foot standing times by age[30,94]

Age	Duration (s) 1-Foot Standing
30 mo	1 (briefly)
36 mo	2
4 y	5

It is valuable to refer children with SNHL whose screening identifies them as being at risk of VD for a comprehensive diagnostic assessment. Evaluation of horizontal canal function with caloric evaluation by videonystagmography, rotary chair and video head impulse testing, and otolithic function assessment by ocular and cervical vestibular evoked myogenic potentials are examples of tests that may be useful in evaluating children. Comprehensive testing to confirm that the vestibular end-organ is indeed the reason for children failing screening of balance and vestibular function is becoming more available due to increasing interest in vestibular testing in the pediatric population.

Developmental Consequences of Vestibular Dysfunction

Sensory deficits impact how children's brains perceive and process sensory information. Deficits of sensory information begin at the affected end-organ, impacting all pathways leading to and including the primary sensory and secondary association cortices of the brain, resulting in anomalies of development.[35–45] Beyond balance, the vestibular system plays an underrecognized role in development of cognition by providing perceptual and visuospatial input important for memory and executive function. Several studies have demonstrated that children with VD reveal deficits in memory and executive function.[46,47] Therefore it is not surprising that an association between VD and poor school performance has been documented.[48] Overall, individuals with VD show poorer performance on all visuospatial tasks specifically including spatial memory, spatial navigation, and mental rotation.[46] A review of the cognitive impact of VD in children suggests that there is likely a critical period in which accurate spatial representations may be developed.[49] Individuals with bilateral VD demonstrate deficits on visuospatial tasks that have correlated neuroanatomically with decreased hippocampal volume.[50]

Children with SNHL also have reduced capacity for serial learning even when information is presented visually, as well as deficits in organizational process and retrieval strategies used in verbal learning and memory tasks of recall of spoken words.[51–53] Early deprivation and the reorganization that happens following rehabilitation may lead to the development of deficits in processes needed for rapid encoding and ordering of recalled information.[52] Our laboratory, which studies hearing and balance in children with SNHL, believes that ongoing functional impairments, such as those described earlier, may be over- or incorrectly attributed to the auditory deficits caused by SNHL, rather than VD. If VD is recognized early, its impact may be reduced through interventive therapy.[54]

Children with unilateral sensorineural hearing loss (UHL) are expected to develop speech perception and spoken language even when profound SNHL is present. It is recognized that this group of children are at academic risk, a situation often attributed to their auditory deficit alone. However, this group of children demonstrate significantly poorer standardized balance scores than normal-hearing peers.[25] More than half of the children with UHL demonstrated VD on vestibular end-organ testing (oto-liths and horizontal canal) with dysfunction most commonly in the ear with SNHL.[55] These children also present with deficits in other domains.[56] For example, difficulties with spatial navigation and localization, which are typically attributed to the auditory deficit, may instead be caused or exacerbated by vestibular and balance impairment, which is common in children with UHL.[25,55] In summary, a portion of the deficits that we observe in children with UHL may be due to combined SNHL-VD deficit as opposed to the SNHL alone.[56,57]

Another important consequence of VD in children with either unilateral or bilateral SNHL is fatigue. Compensation for VD demands use of cognitive resources to accomplish basic tasks such as staying upright or stabilizing vision. Because maintaining postural stability is a priority, spatial and nonspatial tasks are equally impacted by the reduction in cognitive resources created by VD.[58] The use of cognitive resources to maintain balance contributes to fatigue and takes away from the availability of these resources to perform other tasks such as conversing or reading.[46]

Today, many children with SNHL develop listening skills and spoken language by use of amplification and/or cochlear implants (CIs). However, achieving these goals alone does not equal comprehensive rehabilitative success. VD can impact academic and social skills and limit participation in everyday sports and activities. It is often unrecognized or incorrectly attributed to other factors such as personality or cognition. Even when VD is diagnosed, its impact may be missed because long-term outcome measures typically do include the role of balance in daily life. Therefore, the first step to further improve these children's lives is diagnosis of the underlying cause, followed by effective habilitation. Screening of children with SNHL is therefore an important first step.

Cochlear Implantation and Vestibular Dysfunction

Approximately 35% of CI candidates have absent vestibular function before surgery.[2] Of those with normal vestibular function before surgery, the risk of causing total bilateral loss is 2% in children undergoing bilateral implantation.[6,20,59,60] An inability to develop independent ambulation, a concern in the early days of implantation, is not a concern based on several decades of pediatric implant experience. Whether congenital or acquired, VD in CI recipients may be mitigated by vestibular rehabilitation.[61] In addition, children who have received a CI and have VD are more at risk of experiencing failure of the surgically implanted device.[62] This finding, first reported by our research group, is theorized to be related to increased frequency of falls causing microtrauma to the implant.

Management Options Exist and are Expanding

Diagnosis of peripheral VD and understanding its functional impact is valuable in the current management of children with SNHL and is essential to the development of new and improved treatments. Another benefit of diagnosis is parental counseling regarding safety. For example, individuals with bilateral VD may be at increased risk of losing orientation and drown when swimming underwater.[63] There is also increased risk of loss of spatial orientation in the dark due to reduced visual input.

There are different therapeutic approaches for the rehabilitation of children with VD, and for children with deficits of sensory organization and integration, known sequela of VD. At present, habilitation strategies for VD in children primarily focus on adaptation through compensation. This approach may improve balance, but still requires significant central compensation that may contribute to fatigue and limit cognitive resources available for learning.[64–67] Although habilitation may improve balance, head-referenced and gravitational spatial information by the vestibular end-organs is not restored.[68–70] Providing children with this type of sensory input would be highly beneficial. In adults, research on several devices to stabilize balance with vibrotactile stimulation has demonstrated variable benefit.[69,71–74] Technology that provides useful sensory input to improve balance and prevents falls could result in significant functional and safety benefit for children with SNHL.

Sound stimulation of the auditory system provides the brain with information regarding our position in space. Auditory cues have been shown to influence postural alignment.[75,76] A child's ability to maintain balance with diminished vestibular input requires compensatory adjustments.[77,78] Fortunately, children with SNHL-VD can access sound through amplification and/or CI and thereby improve spatial awareness. Several studies have demonstrated that hearing through bilateral CIs may provide children with cues to support balance.[3,5,79] In challenging balance situations, children with SNHL may rely on and integrate senses, including hearing, to stay upright in a way that is different from the strategies of typically developing children.[80] There is also evidence of limited improvement in balance when electric hearing from CI is being used.[3,79,81] Several underlying mechanisms could account for this benefit to balance. First is improved hearing through CI providing additional spatial cues. Second is spread of current from the electrodes within the cochlear turns. Evidence for the latter is growing. Asymptomatic current spread is known to occur in a significant number of CI recipients.[7] It has also been demonstrated that vestibular end-organs including the saccule are stimulated when the CI is activated by sound.[82–84] Our laboratory has also demonstrated vestibular evoked myogenic potentials in response to CI activation and improved patient perception of verticality.[85,86]

Our laboratory is studying a "BalanCI," a CI system that provides information about head position for children with bilateral CI and VD. More stable balance, improved postural control, and reduction in falls have been demonstrated.[87,88] This system may become an important treatment option to improve balance in implanted children.

Another approach to VD is development of implants with electrode arrays designed to directly activate the vestibular system, either with or without stimulation to improve hearing. This approach would be of benefit to individuals with and without SNHL who have functional deficits from VD. This approach is currently being trialed in adults by several research groups.[89–93] Much work is required before such devices come into mainstream clinical practice, particularly for pediatric patients. A prerequisite for use in children will be the early and accurate assessment of the vestibular system.

SUMMARY

VD is common in children with SNHL. The identification of VD is important to understanding potential developmental problems, which may be ameliorated with rehabilitation. Therefore, screening for VD is an important part of the evaluation of children with SNHL. As therapeutic options expand, early and accurate diagnosis of VD will be needed as a foundation for early intervention.

CLINICS CARE POINTS

- Children with SNHL-VD present infrequently with vertigo.
- Bilateral VD in children does not lead to nonambulation.
- Screening for VD in children who present with SNHL is important and necessary.

- One-foot standing (eyes open eyes closed) is an effective screening tool for VD.
- Objective tests of vestibular end-organ function are possible in infants and children.
- Early intervention for VD may reduce functional, neurocognitive, and motor deficits.
- Clinical safety concerns should be relayed to the families of children who present with bilateral VD.

DISCLOSURE

Sharon Cushing: Speaker's Bureau: Interacoustics, Cochlear Corporation.
Royalties: Plural Publishing, Editor: Balance Disorders in the Pediatric Population.
Patent Holder: Patents #: 7041 to 0: Systems and Methods for Balance Stabilization.
Sponsored Research Agreement: Cochlear Americas.

REFERENCES

1. National center for hearing assessment and management. Available at: http://www.infanthearing.org.
2. Cushing SL, Gordon KA, Rutka JA, et al. Vestibular end-organ dysfunction in children with sensorineural hearing loss and cochlear implants: an expanded cohort and etiologic assessment. Otol Neurotol 2013;34(3):422–8.
3. Buchman CA, Joy J, Hodges A, et al. Vestibular effects of cochlear implantation. Laryngoscope 2004;114(10 Pt 2 Suppl 103):1–22.
4. Licameli G, Zhou G, Kenna MA. Disturbance of vestibular function attributable to cochlear implantation in children. Laryngoscope 2009;119(4):740–5.
5. Selz PA, Girardi M, Konrad HR, et al. Vestibular deficits in deaf children. Otolaryngol Head Neck Surg 1996;115(1):70–7.
6. Jacot E, Van Den Abbeele T, Debre HR, et al. VLs pre- and post-cochlear implant in children. Int J Pediatr Otorhinolaryngol 2009;73(2):209–17.
7. Cushing SL, Papsin BC, Gordon KA. Incidence and characteristics of facial nerve stimulation in children with cochlear implants. Laryngoscope 2006;116(10):1787–91.
8. Cushing SLCR, James AL, Papsin BC, et al. The Vestibular Olympics : a test of dynamic balance function in children with cochlear implants. Arch Otorhinolaryngol 2007;134(1):34–8.
9. De Kegel A, Maes L, Baetens T, et al. The influence of a VL on the motor development of hearing-impaired children. Laryngoscope 2012;122(12):2837–43.
10. Huygen PL, van Rijn PM, Cremers CW, et al. The vestibulo-ocular reflex in pupils at a Dutch school for the hearing impaired; findings relating to acquired causes. Int J Pediatr Otorhinolaryngol 1993;25(1–3):39–47.
11. Rapin I. Hypoactive labyrinths and motor development. Clin Pediatr (Phila) 1974;13(11):922–3, 926–9, 934–7.
12. Goldstein R, Landau WM, Kleffner FR. Neurologic assessment of some deaf and aphasic children. Ann Otol Rhinol Laryngol 1958;67(2):468–79.
13. Sandberg LE, Terkildsen K. Caloric tests in deaf children. Arch Otolaryngol 1965;81:350–4.
14. Kaplan SL, Goddard J, Van Kleeck M, et al. Ataxia and deafness in children due to bacterial meningitis. Pediatrics 1981;68(1):8–13.
15. Karjalainen S, Terasvirta M, Karja J, et al. Usher's syndrome type III: ENG findings in four affected and six unaffected siblings. J Laryngol Otol 1985;99(1):43–8.

16. Kumar A, Fishman G, Torok N. Vestibular and auditory function in Usher's syndrome. Ann Otol Rhinol Laryngol 1984;93(6 Pt 1):600–8.

17. Otterstedde CR, Spandau U, Blankenagel A, et al. A new clinical classification for Usher's syndrome based on a new subtype of Usher's syndrome type I. Laryngoscope 2001;111(1):84–6.

18. Samuelson S, Zahn J. Usher's syndrome. Ophthalmic Paediatr Genet 1990; 11(1):71–6.

19. Cushing SL, Papsin BC, Rutka JA, et al. Vestibular end-organ and balance deficits after meningitis and cochlear implantation in children correlate poorly with functional outcome. Otol Neurotol 2009;30(4):488–95.

20. Wiener-Vacher SR, Obeid R, Abou-Elew M. VL after bacterial meningitis delays infant posturomotor development. J Pediatr 2012;161(2):246–51.e1.

21. Dollard SC, Grosse SD, Ross DS. New estimates of the prevalence of neurological and sensory sequelae and mortality associated with congenital cytomegalovirus infection. Rev Med Virol 2007;17(5):355–63.

22. Teissier N, Bernard S, Quesnel S, et al. Audiovestibular consequences of congenital cytomegalovirus infection. Eur Ann Otorhinolaryngol Head Neck Dis 2016;133(6):413–8.

23. Nassar MN, Elmaleh M, Cohen A, et al. Vestibular calcification in a case of congenital cytomegalovirus infection. Otol Neurotol 2015;36(6):e107–9.

24. Bernard S, Wiener-Vacher S, Van Den Abbeele T, et al. Vestibular disorders in children with congenital cytomegalovirus infection. Pediatrics 2015;136(4): e887–95.

25. Wolter NE, Cushing SL, Vilchez-Madrigal LD, et al. Unilateral hearing loss is associated with impaired balance in children: a pilot study. Otol Neurotol 2016;37(10): 1589–95.

26. Kletke S, Batmanabane V, Dai T, et al. The combination of VL and congenital sensorineural hearing loss predisposes patients to ocular anomalies, including Usher syndrome. Clin Genet 2016. https://doi.org/10.1111/cge.12895.

27. luxon L, Pagarkar W. The dizzy child. In: Graham J, Scadding G, Bull P, editors. Pediatric ENT. Springer; 2008. p. 459–78.

28. Ketola S, Niemensivu R, Henttonen A, et al. Somatoform disorders in vertiginous children and adolescents. Int J Pediatr Otorhinolaryngol 2009;73(7):933–6.

29. Cushing SL, MacDonald L, Propst EJ, et al. Successful cochlear implantation in a child with Keratosis, Icthiosis and Deafness (KID) Syndrome and Dandy-Walker malformation. Int J Pediatr Otorhinolaryngol 2008;72(5):693–8.

30. Oyewumi M, Wolter NE, Heon E, et al. Using balance function to screen for VL in children with sensorineural hearing loss and cochlear implants. Otol Neurotol 2016;37(7):926–32.

31. Cushing SL, Papsin BC, Rutka JA, et al. Evidence of vestibular and balance dysfunction in children with profound sensorineural hearing loss using cochlear implants. Laryngoscope 2008;118(10):1814–23.

32. Shumway-Cook A, Woollacott MH. The growth of stability: postural control from a development perspective. J Mot Behav 1985;17(2):131–47.

33. Bruininks R, Bruininks B. BOT-2 Bruininks-Oseretsky test of motor proficiency. 2nd edition. Shoreview (MN): AGS Publishing; 2005. p. 263.

34. Cohen B. Erasmus Darwin's observations on rotation and vertigo. Hum Neurobiol 1984;3(3):121–8.

35. Pienkowski M, Harrison RV. Tone frequency maps and receptive fields in the developing chinchilla auditory cortex. J Neurophysiol 2005;93(1):454–66.

36. Pienkowski M, Harrison RV. Tone responses in core versus belt auditory cortex in the developing chinchilla. J Comp Neurol 2005;492(1):101–9.

37. Mount RJ, Takeno S, Wake M, et al. Carboplatin ototoxicity in the chinchilla: lesions of the vestibular sensory epithelium. Acta Otolaryngol Suppl 1995; 519:60–5.

38. Harrison RV, Ibrahim D, Mount RJ. Plasticity of tonotopic maps in auditory midbrain following partial cochlear damage in the developing chinchilla. Exp Brain Res 1998;123(4):449–60.

39. Brown TA, Harrison RV. Neuronal responses in chinchilla auditory cortex after postnatal exposure to frequency-modulated tones. Hear Res 2011; 275(1–2):8–16.

40. Brown TA, Harrison RV. Postnatal development of neuronal responses to frequency-modulated tones in chinchilla auditory cortex. Brain Res 2010;1309: 29–39.

41. Brown TA, Harrison RV. Responses of neurons in chinchilla auditory cortex to frequency-modulated tones. J Neurophysiol 2009;101(4):2017–29.

42. Yamazaki H, Easwar V, Polonenko MJ, et al. Cortical hemispheric asymmetries are present at young ages and further develop into adolescence. Hum Brain Mapp 2018;39(2):941–54.

43. Jiwani S, Papsin BC, Gordon KA. Early unilateral cochlear implantation promotes mature cortical asymmetries in adolescents who are deaf. Hum Brain Mapp 2016; 37(1):135–52.

44. Jiwani S, Papsin BC, Gordon KA. Central auditory development after long-term cochlear implant use. Clin Neurophysiol 2013;124(9):1868–80.

45. Gordon KA, Jiwani S, Papsin BC. Benefits and detriments of unilateral cochlear implant use on bilateral auditory development in children who are deaf. Front Psychol 2013;4:719.

46. Bigelow RT, Agrawal Y. Vestibular involvement in cognition: Visuospatial ability, attention, executive function, and memory. J Vestib Res 2015;25(2):73–89.

47. Beer J, Kronenberger WG, Castellanos I, et al. Executive functioning skills in preschool-age children with cochlear implants. J Speech Lang Hear Res 2014; 57(4):1521–34.

48. Franco ES, Panhoca I. Vestibular function in children underperforming at school. Braz J Otorhinolaryngol 2008;74(6):815–25.

49. Wiener-Vacher SR, Hamilton DA, Wiener SI. Vestibular activity and cognitive development in children: perspectives. Front Integr Neurosci 2013;7:92.

50. Brandt T, Schautzer F, Hamilton DA, et al. VL causes hippocampal atrophy and impaired spatial memory in humans. Brain 2005;128(Pt 11):2732–41.

51. Pisoni DB. Cognitive factors and cochlear implants: some thoughts on perception, learning, and memory in speech perception. Ear Hear 2000;21(1):70–8.

52. Pisoni DB, Kronenberger WG, Chandramouli SH, et al. Learning and memory processes following cochlear implantation: the missing piece of the puzzle. Front Psychol 2016;7:493.

53. Conway CM, Bauernschmidt A, Huang SS, et al. Implicit statistical learning in language processing: word predictability is the key. Cognition 2010;114(3):356–71.

54. Cohen HS, Kimball KT. Improvements in path integration after vestibular rehabilitation. J Vestib Res 2002;12(1):47–51.

55. Sokolov M, Gordon KA, Polonenko M, et al. Vestibular and balance function is often impaired in children with profound unilateral sensorineural hearing loss. Hear Res 2019;372:52–61.

56. Lieu JE, Tye-Murray N, Fu Q. Longitudinal study of children with unilateral hearing loss. Laryngoscope 2012;122(9):2088–95.

57. Bess FH, Tharpe AM. Unilateral hearing impairment in children. Pediatrics 1984; 74(2):206–16.

58. Yardley L, Papo D, Bronstein A, et al. Attentional demands of continuously monitoring orientation using vestibular information. Neuropsychologia 2002;40(4): 373–83.

59. Wiener Vacher S, Petrof N, Francois M, et al. Impact of cochear implant of vestibular function in children and decision betweentwo steps or one step bilateral implant. Paper presented at 12th European Symposium on Pediatric Cochlear Implants; 18–21 June 2015; Toulouse, France.

60. Thierry B, Blanchard M, Leboulanger N, et al. Cochlear implantation and vestibular function in children. Int J Pediatr Otorhinolaryngol 2015;79(2):101–4.

61. Wolter NE, Gordon KA, Campos J, et al. Impact of the sensory environment on balance in children with bilateral cochleovestibular loss. Hearing Res 2021;400: 108132–4.

62. Wolter NE, Gordon KA, Papsin BC, et al. Vestibular and balance impairment contributes to cochlear implant failure in children. Otol Neurotol 2015;36(6):1029–34.

63. Verhagen WI, Huygen PL, Horstink MW. Familial congenital vestibular areflexia. J Neurol Neurosurg Psychiatry 1987;50(7):933–5.

64. Effgen SK. Effect of an exercise program on the static balance of deaf children. Phys Ther 1981;61(6):873–7.

65. Medeiros IR, Bittar RS, Pedalini ME, et al. Vestibular rehabilitation therapy in children. Otol Neurotol 2005;26(4):699–703.

66. Crowe TK, Horak FB. Motor proficiency associated with vestibular deficits in children with hearing impairments. Phys Ther 1988;68(10):1493–9.

67. Gronski MP, Bogan KE, Kloeckner J, et al. Childhood toxic stress: a community role in health promotion for occupational therapists. Am J Occup Ther 2013; 67(6):e148–53.

68. Barra J, Marquer A, Joassin R, et al. Humans use internal models to construct and update a sense of verticality. Brain 2010;133(Pt 12):3552–63.

69. Horak FB. Postural compensation for VL and implications for rehabilitation. Restor Neurol Neurosci 2010;28(1):57–68.

70. Gaertner C, Bucci MP, Obeid R, et al. Subjective visual vertical and postural performance in healthy children. PLoS One 2013;8(11):e79623.

71. Wong AM, Lee MY, Kuo JK, et al. The development and clinical evaluation of a standing biofeedback trainer. J Rehabil Res Dev 1997;34(3):322–7.

72. Kentala E, Vivas J, Wall C 3rd. Reduction of postural sway by use of a vibrotactile balance prosthesis prototype in subjects with vestibular deficits. Ann Otol Rhinol Laryngol 2003;112(5):404–9.

73. Dozza M, Chiari L, Horak FB. Audio-biofeedback improves balance in patients with bilateral VL. Arch Phys Med Rehabil 2005;86(7):1401–3.

74. Dozza M, Chiari L, Chan B, et al. Influence of a portable audio-biofeedback device on structural properties of postural sway. J Neuroeng Rehabil 2005;2:13.

75. Lackner JR. The role of posture in sound localization. Q J Exp Psychol 1974; 26(2):235–51.

76. Lackner JR. Changes in auditory localization during body tilt. Acta Otolaryngol 1974;77(1):19–28.

77. Kaga K. Vestibular compensation in infants and children with congenital and acquired VL in both ears. Int J Pediatr Otorhinolaryngol 1999;49(3):215–24.

78. Suarez H, Angeli S, Suarez A, et al. Balance sensory organization in children with profound hearing loss and cochlear implants. Int J Pediatr Otorhinolaryngol 2007; 71(4):629–37.
79. Cushing SL, Chia R, James AL, et al. A test of static and dynamic balance function in children with cochlear implants: the vestibular olympics. Arch Otolaryngol Head Neck Surg 2008;134(1):34–8.
80. Mazaheryazdi M, Moossavi A, Sarrafzadah J, et al. Study of the effects of hearing on static and dynamic postural function in children using cochlear implants. Int J Pediatr Otorhinolaryngol 2017;100:18–22.
81. Eisenberg LS, Nelson JR, House WF. Effects of the single-electrode cochlear implant on the vestibular system of the profoundly deaf adult. Ann Otol Rhinol Laryngol Suppl 1982;91(2 Pt 3):47–54.
82. Black FO, Wall C 3rd, O'Leary DP, et al. Galvanic disruption of vestibulospinal postural control by cochlear implant devices. J Otolaryngol 1978;7(6):519–27.
83. Bance ML, O'Driscoll M, Giles E, et al. Vestibular stimulation by multichannel cochlear implants. Laryngoscope 1998;108(2):291–4.
84. Ito J. Influence of the multichannel cochlear implant on vestibular function. Otolaryngol Head Neck Surg 1998;118(6):900–2.
85. Parkes WJ, Gnanasegaram JJ, Cushing SL, et al. Vestibular evoked myogenic potential testing as an objective measure of vestibular stimulation with cochlear implants. Laryngoscope 2017;127(2):E75–81.
86. Gnanasegaram JJ, Parkes WJ, Cushing SL, et al. Stimulation from cochlear implant electrodes assists with recovery from asymmetric perceptual tilt: evidence from the subjective visual vertical test. Front Integr Neurosci 2016;10:32.
87. Wolter NE, Gordon KA, Campos JL, et al. BalanCI: head-referenced cochlear implant stimulation improves balance in children with bilateral cochleoVL. Audiol Neurootol 2020;25(1–2):60–71.
88. Cushing SL, Pothier D, Hughes C, et al. Providing auditory cues to improve stability in children who are deaf. Laryngoscope 2012;122(Suppl 4):S101–2.
89. Della Santina CC, Migliaccio AA, Patel AH. A multichannel semicircular canal neural prosthesis using electrical stimulation to restore 3-d vestibular sensation. IEEE Trans Biomed Eng 2007;54(6 Pt 1):1016–30.
90. Fridman GY, Della Santina CC. Progress toward development of a multichannel vestibular prosthesis for treatment of bilateral vestibular deficiency. Anat Rec (Hoboken) 2012;295(11):2010–29.
91. Rubinstein JT, Nie K, Bierer S, et al. Signal processing for a vestibular neurostimulator. Conf Proc IEEE Eng Med Biol Soc 2010;2010:6247.
92. Phillips JO, Shepherd SJ, Nowack AL, et al. Longitudinal performance of a vestibular prosthesis as assessed by electrically evoked compound action potential recording. Conf Proc IEEE Eng Med Biol Soc 2012;2012:6128–31.
93. Bierer SM, Ling L, Nie K, et al. Auditory outcomes following implantation and electrical stimulation of the semicircular canals. *Hear Res* May 2012;287(1–2):51–6.
94. Shea S. Chapter 5. *Developmental assessment.* In: Goldbloom RB, editor. Pediatric clinical skills. 2nd edition. Churchill Livingstone; 1997. p. 95–118.

Moving?

Make sure your subscription moves with you!

To notify us of your new address, find your **Clinics Account Number** (located on your mailing label above your name), and contact customer service at:

Email: journalscustomerservice-usa@elsevier.com

800-654-2452 (subscribers in the U.S. & Canada)
314-447-8871 (subscribers outside of the U.S. & Canada)

Fax number: 314-447-8029

Elsevier Health Sciences Division
Subscription Customer Service
3251 Riverport Lane
Maryland Heights, MO 63043

*To ensure uninterrupted delivery of your subscription, please notify us at least 4 weeks in advance of move.

Printed and bound by CPI Group (UK) Ltd, Croydon, CR0 4YY

03/10/2024

01040470-0016